got teens?

LOGAN LEVKOFF PhD
and JENNIFER WIDER MD

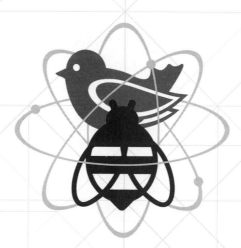

got teens?

The Doctor Moms' Guide to
Sexuality, Social Media and
Other Adolescent Realities

SEAL PRESS

Got Teens?
The Doctor Moms' Guide to Sexuality, Social Media, and Other Adolescent Realities

Published by
Seal Press
A Member of the Perseus Books Group
1700 Fourth Street
Berkeley, California

Library of Congress Cataloging-in-Publication Data

Levkoff, Logan.
  Got teens? : the doctor moms' guide to sexuality, social media and other
adolescent realities / Logan Levkoff, Ph.D. and Jennifer Wider, M.D.
    pages cm

  ISBN 978-1-58005-506-2 (pbk.)
  1. Health behavior in adolescence. 2. Parent and teenager. 3. Mothers
and sons. 4. Adolescent psychology. I. Wider, Jennifer. II. Title.
  RJ47.53.L48 2014
  613'.0433--dc23

                          2013040092

Cover design by Jeff Miller, Faceout Studio
Interior design by meganjonesdesign.com

Printed in the United States of America
9 8 7 6 5 4 3 2 1

Distributed by Publishers Group West

To parents, relatives, caregivers, and friends
who are helping children through adolescence
empowered with knowledge and self-esteem,
surrounded by love and understanding

CONTENTS

introduction

Who Are the Doctor Moms?

(AND, MORE IMPORTANTLY, WHY YOU NEED THIS BOOK)

DR. JENA WIDER

I am on the edge, straddling two worlds, and my anxiety is rising. As I write this, my ten-year-old daughter has but weeks left in elementary school, a place where she has been sheltered, looked after by teachers, recess monitors, and even the bus driver. This preteen world seems much safer than what lies ahead.

My own memories of middle school are hazy, though I remember being nervous, having books knocked out of my hands, and also being expected to act grown-up. But what about the world my daughter is entering? She, too, may be shoved around in the halls, and she, too, may be nervous. But her world also seems more fraught; it is one filled with gadgets and images that heighten both my anxiety and hers: iPhones, texting, YouTube, the Kardashians.

It makes my head spin. I have spent the entirety of motherhood trying to protect my daughter from every scrape, bruise, and bump, trying to shield her from every unkind word or mean-spirited jab, and now that she is entering middle school, I can only hope that I have helped her harness a sense of independence, a sense of confidence, and the ability to make good, healthy decisions. My anxiety stems from a nagging fear: Have I in fact accomplished this as a parent?

As a physician and educator, on the other hand, I know what to expect. I have given hundreds of talks to parents on adolescent development, health, and sexuality education. In the questions I hear from parents, I sense desperation in their voices as they look for guidance and advice on how to approach their children or even initiate a conversation about the tough issues sure to arise in the near future. One mom, for example, had walked in on her son masturbating and had no clue if or how to talk to him. Another mom was worried that her fourth-grade daughter's unibrow was so unsightly that the girl would be teased. Her daughter, on the other hand, was oblivious. When is the right age for grooming and beauty treatments, and would calling attention to this girl's eyebrows actually make her more self-conscious? These are but two of the many similar questions I hear all the time that capture parents' anxiety about handling these situations in this new era of their child's development the right way.

What these parents are really asking is: Will I be able to communicate the important facts and lessons about puberty and adolescence to my children (who seem more interested in texting than in talking)? Will I be able to protect my children from embarrassment—or worse?

What I want to tell them is: Yes, yes, yes. You may have to open yourself up to unfamiliar and perhaps uncomfortable conversations at first, but it will get easier. Arm yourself with correct, solid information, and really think through your communication strategies. Because if you're anxious, you may be tempted to not even deal with these issues at all. More important, what I want to tell parents is that such conversations shouldn't even be "issues"— they should simply be a normal part of growing up. At the same time, though I am armed with these facts because I am a doctor, I am also a mother, and I totally get it.

DR. LOGAN LEVKOFF

Although my children are years away from middle school, they ask many of the same questions that older kids ask. Sure, part of that curiosity comes from the fact that because I am a sexuality educator, they are the consummate sex-ed guinea pigs: if they ask a question, they always get an answer. As such, they've learned to ask lots of questions. But they don't ask just because they are my children (as much as I'd like to take all the credit). They ask because all of us are curious about our bodies and about that societally forbidden word: *sex*. While younger children and older adolescents may have identical questions, they ask for different reasons, obviously. Older children are curious about sex and relationships and bodies because those concepts relate directly to them. Younger children are just trying to decode language and make sense of the world around them.

Even though my children are not pubescent yet, I am acutely aware of the need for them (and their friends) to develop a healthy, positive sense of self. I see it going on in the classrooms regularly: grotesque slang references to body parts; language that perpetuates a vicious sexual double standard; jokes (often inadvertent ones) about being "gay." I cringe at the thought of others sabotaging the work that I've been doing with my son and daughter since they were born; however, I know that our ongoing conversations will always be a good litmus test to identify the competing (and questionable) information and values they encounter.

But, like Jena's, my two worlds are constantly colliding. As an educator who teaches schoolchildren, I am on the front lines of adolescent angst and am frustrated that my time with my students is limited to a forty-five-minute class period. But as a parent, I know that sexuality education doesn't take place only in schools. It also goes on daily in our homes and in carpool lines, because parents are the primary sexuality educators for our children. We are the ones who tell our children that they are beautiful no matter what, that rejection hurts, that they will eventually develop—or that their peers will catch up. We do the heavy lifting. What we teach our children about puberty, sex, and critical thinking directly impacts the choices they make. And we can't opt out of this. It's our job, and we can do that job very well.

But that's not exactly what happens, right? We stick our heads in the sand and pretend that if we don't acknowledge it, it won't happen. Or we rely on teachers to do it, but what happens when our children have a question, or an issue arises, and they are no longer sitting in their sex education class—if they even get one of those at all?

Sure, this may sound harsh, but it's said with love. Seriously. My own girlfriends have the same issues that most parents have— they don't know what to say or how to say it—until they sit down with me. I've spent many unbillable hours with them (typically over glasses of wine or margaritas), encouraging them to talk and empowering them with support and guidance.

THE DOCTOR MOMS

So here we are. Let us be your friends. Imagine us sitting next to you on a banquette at a restaurant somewhere. We're laughing, we're talking, we're sharing stories, and we're giving you the facts and support that you need to tackle challenging subjects. That's who we are for the people in our lives; we want to do the same for you.

Not only are middle school-age children entering a new world with many unchecked influences from peers and the media, but they are leaving an old world in which we—their parents—intimately know every angle and curve of our children's bodies. All of a sudden, these children whom we raised want privacy for those bodies. And we are caught between the emotional reality that our babies are growing up and the desire to (quite appropriately) respect the emotional and physical privacy that our middle schoolers crave. Understandably, this anxiety can lead to inaction—and even to inadvertent ignorance.

Study after study has suggested that good, honest, open communication between parent and child positively influences a child's ability to make responsible choices. So where is the line between this openness and privacy? Pubescent children likely crave both. Yet many of us don't realize that we should begin talking to our children about physical and sexual development much earlier than we do. In addition, many of the parents we talk to don't follow through on the small openings their children provide and instead wind up cutting short communication at essential, pivotal times. In short, many parents have lost the ability to operate on instinct, so they don't say anything.

Why don't we say anything? At the heart of it, we're probably embarrassed. We remember many less-than-ideal moments, including these two:

Logan was the first girl in her class to wear a bra (and get her period). When she was in sixth grade, a boy named Jeffrey (whom she despised) tried to grab her breasts. Logan pushed him off her—he never even came close to them—but he told her entire class that she had "soccer-ball tits." She was eleven, and she was mortified.

The summer Jena got her period, she was turning thirteen and attending a coed sports camp. Her mom told her that it was okay to swim while menstruating—no reason to stress. So, like any other adolescent girl, she put on her bathing suit, wrapped an Always pad with wings around the bottom of the suit, and jumped off the ten-foot diving board into the deep end. She came up first, followed by her pad, which was the size of a personal pan pizza. Instead of disowning the incident, she grabbed the pad and quit camp the next day, humiliated.

MAYBE THIS KIND of embarrassing moment for you was getting an erection while giving a class presentation or having a bra snapped or developing a huge whitehead on school-picture day. It's no wonder that when our children reach puberty, we feel their own awkwardness so acutely. And when our memories of that time in our own lives continue to stand out for us, it can be difficult for us to approach our children's questions about their development and sexuality with openness and ease.

While it would be nice if our children never had to experience a single embarrassing moment in their lives, that isn't going to happen anytime soon. Adolescence is chock-full of mortifying moments for children—not to mention parents who may flounder when confronted with a from-left-field question about, say, Brazilian bikini waxes. But, when armed with up-to-date, accurate information and a few strategies for handling the tough conversations, we have the opportunity (and, dare we say it, responsibility) to give our children the information and understanding they need to survive the precarious, precious time that is puberty. (Imagine how different your experience would have been if you had been equipped with solid, positive, loving information, instead of relying on the unchanged-since-1975 puberty-and-sex video that that you got in that sad excuse for a health class in the fifth grade.)

Besides, we like to think that we are different today. Maybe we could call it cool parenting. Maybe we could call it new-world parenting. We suppose it doesn't really matter what label we slap on it, though. Our parenting responsibilities are the same; it's the world that looks—that *is*—different.

This point hit home for Logan one day when she was with her children in her car, listening to the radio, and "Mother Mother," by Tracy Bonham, came through the speakers. In her previous life, before she had children and a slew of grown-up responsibilities, Logan sang this very song in a band at a dive bar in Queens, New York. She still remembers the lyrics perfectly: "When you sent me off to see the world, were you scared that I might get hurt? Would I try a little tobacco? Would I keep on hiking up my skirt?" Back then it seemed like the perfect song of rebellion, a means of saying: *Screw you! I'm on my own. And I'm, well, sort of fine about that.* As a twenty-one-year-old, Logan could belt it out and imagine singing it to parents all over the world. Now she makes sense of it differently.

As she looked at her children rocking out in the backseat, she wondered if what Bonham sang about her own mother rings true for Logan as a mother today. Sure, she is scared that her children might get hurt, but that's about it. She definitely doesn't worry about her daughter hiking up her skirt (actually, she expects it); as for trying tobacco, she accepts that there are things in life that her children will try, against their (and Logan's) better judgment. However, she hopes that the way she talks to her kids during their formative years can help them to reduce any harm that comes from experimentation.

It's this type of reality-based parenting that we need today. No more judgments. We need to listen, we need to talk honestly, and we need to remember that we were young once, too.

1

Puberty, Body Development, and Anatomy

PART 1:
PUBERTY AND THE BODY

S O, YOUR ONCE-ANGELIC, patient, and loving child has recently turned into a werewolf: she snaps at you, loses her cool easily, and goes right to her room when she gets home. When you ask, "How was school?" her response is barely audible. Sometimes she's fine and you get glimpses of the little girl with pigtails who used to hold your hand while watching *Dora the Explorer*; other times you barely recognize her. She's moody, emotional, angry, and hard to talk to; you feel at a loss. Trust us, you are not alone. Millions of parents before you have dealt with this, and millions of parents after you will, too. Your child is going through puberty.

From a biological standpoint, puberty is a progression of physical changes that turn your child's body into the body of an adult who is capable of sexual reproduction. It involves several stages that occur over a number of years. The onset of puberty can vary from person to person but always starts when the pituitary gland, a bean-shaped gland that sits at the base of the brain, releases special chemicals, called hormones, that signal different parts of the body. For boys, the hormones travel through the bloodstream and tell the testes to begin making testosterone; for girls, the hormones take the same path through the bloodstream but tell the ovaries to start producing estrogen. These sex hormones, estrogen and testosterone, cause most of the changes that your child will experience during puberty, including voice changes; breast development; facial, underarm, and pubic hair growth; genital growth; and menstruation.

But it's not just their bodies that are affected; it's their minds, too. The process can also have a dramatic effect on your child's psychosocial and emotional development. And that's why frequent mood swings, excessive emotional reactions, and a wide variety of feelings—like confusion, sadness, and anger—can play a central role.

We've given you a quick overview of the biology of puberty, but, as we all know, the physical changes are only one part of this transitional process. So take a deep breath, because this is going to take a while.

If you can manage the time and the emotional cost of a trip down memory lane, this is a good moment to bring out the old photographs. Yes, you know what we're talking about—those awful pictures of you with the mouthful of braces and the shaggy-dog haircut (okay, that was Logan in fifth grade). Put yourself back in that time when everything felt overwhelming. Your body was changing, your emotions were running amok, and it seemed like your parents just didn't understand you.

Remember those days? Well, now *you* are the parent who doesn't understand. So do yourself a favor and let your children know that they are not the first (or the last) to feel this way. And don't just tell them that you understand—*show* them. Yes, show them those awful photos. Take out your old yearbooks so that they can see how many millions of young people before them fumbled around during this time—including their parents.

Seriously, being perceived as human is half the battle for you. So, while you may want to yell and scream and lock up your kids until puberty ends, that's just not realistic. It's time to play nice and, in this case, play to their sensitivities, because whether you like it or not, you've been there. (And if you happen to be a peri-menopausal woman, you are probably currently experiencing these highs and lows, too. Use that to your advantage.)

Try to relax; it will keep things in perspective. In the meantime, we'll help you answer some of the most common questions raised by parents of adolescents.

1 Zits can be gross. How can I help my child get rid of them?

Ask a bunch of pubescent kids what the most annoying part of puberty is, and many will tell you that it's acne. No one likes to get pimples, but almost everyone gets them at one time or another, during puberty and beyond. Acne is caused by the same hormones responsible for the other changes that your child will experience during puberty.

As the level of puberty hormones increases in the body, the production of oil, known as sebum, increases as well. When sebum builds up to higher levels, it can block the pores or ducts of the skin. Dirt, bacteria, and dead skin cells can then build up in the pores and cause pimples to form.

There are many different types of acne, and it can occur in varying degrees of severity, depending on the person. If the top of the blocked pore closes and protrudes out from the skin, a white-head forms. If the pore gets blocked but stays open, dirt and debris can accumulate and result in a blackhead. Acne that is deeper in the skin and thereby causes hard, painful cysts is known as cystic acne.

INTERESTING FACTS ABOUT ACNE

:• More than 75 percent of adolescents, or three in four, will experience acne at some point during puberty, according to statistics from the US National Library of Medicine in Bethesda, Maryland.

:• Acne most commonly shows up on the face and shoulders but can also appear on the trunk, arms, legs, and buttocks.

:• Boys are more likely to get severe acne than girls.

:• Severe acne is often an inherited condition, so if you suffered from it as a teenager, your child is more likely to experience it during puberty as well. (Hey, remember what we said earlier about sharing your experiences? Here's a perfect example. If you had acne as a teen and haven't burned those pictures, take them out!)

:• Acne can flare up during different times in a girl's (and woman's) menstrual cycle, especially in the week or so leading up to menstruation.

:• Recent research disproves the link between chocolate, nuts, and greasy foods and acne, but diets high in refined sugar may play a role in skin issues for some people.

Acne can be very disconcerting for your child; they wouldn't be the first kid to want to hide under the bed to avoid a middle school dance. Even a mild case can send your child into a tailspin of self-consciousness, so definitely take their concerns seriously.

The good news is that there are preventive measures that you can encourage your child to take to lower their risk of acne breakouts. Keep in mind the factors that trigger acne, including poor hygiene, stress, cosmetic and hair products, certain medications, humidity, and sweating.

Encourage your child to:

- **Develop a good cleansing program** that consists of washing their face each morning and night with gentle soap and water.

- **Stop touching their face.** Hands are full of bacteria and can trigger an acne breakout.

- **Keep their hair away from the face** and avoid hair products (like hairspray and gel) that can clog pores.

- **Change and discard razors frequently,** especially if they are having facial breakouts.

- **Try over-the-counter medications,** like salicylic acid and benzoyl peroxide, which may help lower the incidence of acne.

- **Bring in the professionals.** See a dermatologist if a daily cleansing routine and over-the-counter medications aren't working. The doctor can prescribe stronger medications that help keep acne under control.

Here's the thing about acne: It looks awful, but young people incorrectly associate it with being dirty or greasy, even when they are meticulous about washing their face and body.

Everyone will have a pimple (or ten) at some point in their life. We still get them now. It's never fun, but, well, things happen. But in addition to your child's self-consciousness about the way they look, there is also the issue of how the outside world perceives them. Your child's face is the one thing that people get to see instantly. And if they aren't happy, they are going to want to hide their face from the world. What we need to do is give them the best tools available for bringing that face back into the open.

And they're not alone. Even kids' favorite celebrities are becoming more public about their tales of acne-ridden skin. Katy Perry and Justin Bieber are just two examples of pop stars who have appeared in advertisements for acne treatments, complete with photos of their broken-out faces. While we don't always buy into what celebrities say or do, in this case we think it's brave of them to put their "worst" face forward.

Though it may seem silly for our children to care about what their favorite stars think, they do. They want some way to connect with their idols. Showing them that the people they admire also deal with acne may be a helpful way for you to connect with your kids.

❷ Why can't my child sleep?

Getting a good night's sleep is particularly important during puberty because the body is changing and growing rapidly. During this time, children need at least nine hours of sleep every night, but getting that much can be a challenge. Thanks to all those hormones, an adolescent's body clock shifts during this time and makes it harder for them to wake up in the morning, even if they have had nine hours of peaceful rest. Many kids report that they don't start to feel sleepy until later but that they then need to sleep in. This is usually impossible on the weekdays because of school. Others report that they wake up once or twice during the night, instead of sleeping straight through to the morning. As a result of these changes, many kids walk around chronically sleep-deprived.

Fatigue and exhaustion are issues for people of all ages, but they can have unique consequences for developing adolescents. Children who are sleep-deprived often have a harder time concentrating and remembering things, which can negatively impact their schoolwork. Sleep deprivation can also lessen a person's ability to deal with everyday stresses. Middle school is a time of anxiety for many students, a delicate act of balancing new academic challenges and social pressure. Add sleep deprivation to the mix, and kids often feel overwhelmed, which can in turn exacerbate the existing irritability and moodiness that come along with puberty. A chronic lack of sleep can also lower teens' immune response, making them more vulnerable to getting sick.

We all know how tough insomnia can be. Try to share a story or two with your child to let them know that it's something we all have to deal with from time to time. Nothing bad will happen to them, other than their feeling sleepier than usual. Their bodies will most likely make up for lost sleep over the next few days. Jena remembers staying up late to study for a midterm exam in tenth grade; when she finally went to bed, it was well past 1:00 AM. But she couldn't fall asleep and became more and more stressed watching the clock. She finally got up after a long struggle and watched one too many *Family Ties* reruns. She ended up doing fine on the exam, despite the extra stress, and slept like a baby the next night.

One of the best things you can do as a parent is to encourage proper sleep habits. Helping your child maximize the amount of sleep they get can lessen the stress cycle and promote their ability to manage the academic and social challenges they may face. Here are a few tips to keep in mind:

:• Establish a routine: Your child should go to bed and wake up at roughly the same time every night and morning. Studies show that changing the schedule too often can deregulate their internal clock.

:• Avoid caffeine late in the day. For some people, this means no caffeinated products—which include coffee, tea, certain soft drinks, and chocolate—after 3:00 PM. For others, it can be later.

:• Exercise is great, but not too close to bedtime. Working out too close to bedtime can interfere with a good night's sleep because the endorphins pumping through your child's body will rev them up.

:• Make their room a dark, calm boy or girl cave. Rooms
filled with electronics like iPads, Xboxes, computers, and televisions can interfere with their ability to
sleep. Recent research underscores this point and even
highlights the fact that the light some of these gadgets'
screens emit can pose a significant challenge to sleeping soundly. In addition, news stories, reality-TV shows,
and other dramatic or suspense-filled programs can
overstimulate your child and hinder their slumber.

If your child can't fall asleep, dissuade them from watching
the clock. There's nothing worse than seeing the clock turn from
1:05 to 1:07 to 1:12 AM; it causes a tremendous amount of an-
ticipatory anxiety, which further exacerbates the problem. If they
haven't fallen asleep after thirty to forty minutes, encourage them
to get up and read or meditate and try again, rather than lie there
tossing and turning.

**③ My daughter is attracted to a classmate whom she
used to think was annoying. Is that normal?**

We don't control whom we are attracted to, and while it would
be far easier to have a crush on the kid who has been nice to you
since kindergarten, life isn't always so convenient. Instead, our
first crushes are often on the people who drive us crazy. Who

did it for you? Logan was always partial to the overly obnoxious boys—the ones who were far from nice and somewhat like mini-Neanderthals. (When she was older, that changed to the people who were just arrogant and egomaniacal. What can she say? She turned out okay.)

We are attracted to people for all different reasons. There is no single definition of *attractive*. Thankfully, that's what makes life exciting. You never know whom you are going to wind up falling for. So, instead of worrying about your daughter's inconvenient crush, use this as an opportunity to think about starting fresh and encouraging her to see all of her peers in an entirely new light.

4 My child can't stop touching himself; I recently caught him masturbating to a catalog that came in the mail. Is this normal?

The first time a parent catches a child "in the act" can be unsettling. It is the most obvious sign that your child is a sexual being. (By the way, they've been sexual beings since birth; it just hasn't been noticeable to you until now.) What should you do? Talk to your son about it? Leave it alone? Please believe us when we tell you that you are certainly not alone in this discovery. In one study of teenage boys, three in four admitted to masturbating, but there's this old joke that 99 percent of teenage boys masturbate and the other 1 percent lie about it.

From a medical perspective, masturbation is normal and harmless. It can release sexual tension, stress, and anxiety. Some studies even reveal masturbation to be effective in strengthening the immune system, improving prostate-gland function, and lowering the risk of prostate infections. Masturbation can also relieve menstrual cramps and has also been touted as a mood booster. It is also a natural sleep aid. Masturbation teaches us about our bodies, how they function, and their innate capacity for pleasure, all of which are essential to good sexual health. In short, self-stimulation is a safe and normal part of sexual exploration, with many benefits.

From a cultural and educational perspective, the conversation about masturbation is typically a gendered one. Often we talk about masturbation through a male lens, as if it is only boys who explore their bodies. This is certainly not the case, and the question posed above could easily have been about someone's daughter. Both males and females are curious about their bodies and what types of pleasure they are capable of producing. If we speak about masturbation as only a "boy's" behavior, we inadvertently tell our daughters that if they do touch their genitals (or want to), there is something wrong with them. If that's the case, girls will feel shameful and guilty about their bodies and desire. This negative self-image can impact how and if girls speak up about pleasure, protection, and equality in their relationships. We want our daughters to feel as empowered by their bodies as our sons do.

So, even though masturbation is a completely safe and healthy sexual exploration for both boys and girls, it nevertheless is often considered a "private" topic, and many parents have a difficult time discussing it with their children. Here's a helpful script for parents who stumble upon their child in the act:

"I know that you're going to want to explore your body and that you may not want to talk to me about it. Just know that it is completely normal. You are growing up, and we will respect your privacy, if you want it. If you have questions about masturbation but don't want to talk to us about it, you can talk to older siblings, friends, or your doctor, especially if you have any concerns. Doctors have seen and heard just about everything, so don't feel embarrassed; they've probably heard it all before."

By the same token, it's important to know that constant or obsessive masturbation *can* be the sign of a problem, so if you find that your child is masturbating compulsively and getting sore or irritated because of it, or if masturbation is getting in the way of their normal daily activities, it may be time to discuss this issue with a doctor.

⑤ Why are my child's skin and hair so oily? She hates it.

Those same hormones that contribute to acne in your child promote the production of extra oil on the hair and skin during puberty. Specifically, a hormone called dihydrotestosterone (DHT), which is a byproduct of testosterone metabolism, serves to regulate oil production in the body. Glands, called sebaceous glands, lie under the skin's surface and produce sebum, or oil, which lubricate and protect the skin and hair. With the onset of puberty, the production of DHT accelerates and causes these glands to go into overdrive and produce extra oil, which can make the face and hair look shiny and greasy.

DHT production increases in both boys and girls during puberty. In girls, the production of DHT can fluctuate during the month, which is why some girls experience oily skin in the days leading up to menstruation. The level of DHT in the body varies from person to person, and that's why some adolescents will notice this more than others. Some studies indicate a genetic predisposition to oily hair and skin, so if you suffered from excess oil as a child, your child may be more likely to encounter this issue during puberty. In addition, steroid use can increase the level of DHT in the body.

Keep in mind that oily skin and hair can be upsetting for your child. They may feel embarrassed or self-conscious or worry that people think they have poor hygiene habits. The good news is that excess oil can be managed.

FOR OILY SKIN:

:• Use a mild cleanser (some are designed specifically for oily skin) with lukewarm water both morning and night.

:• If your child is using cosmetics, encourage oil-free, water-based varieties only.

:• Avoid the use of facial moisturizers, which can exacerbate the problem.

:• If your child's face gets oily midday, pack oil-blotting paper in their backpack that they can use in the bathroom between classes.

:• If acne breakouts occur due to the extra oil production, follow the advice in the acne question earlier in this chapter (page 14).

FOR OILY HAIR:

:• Encourage daily use of a shampoo designed for oily hair.

:• Use only conditioners that are oil-free or designed specifically for oily hair.

:• Use conditioner sparingly, and apply a small amount to the ends of the hair, rather than the top of the scalp, where greasiness can worsen.

:• Don't overbrush hair; doing so can transfer oil from the scalp into the hair itself.

6 My child smells. How can I let her know?

When your child reaches puberty, they may begin to notice a funky smell coming from their armpits or groin area. Body odor is a normal part of puberty and is caused by the hormones that are triggering all of the other changes in the body. Some kids notice a stronger odor coming from one armpit than from the other; this is normal, too. The other armpit usually catches up over time.

During puberty, the hormones increase the output of sweat glands. There are lots of these glands under the arms and in the groin area, so these areas in particular get sweaty and smelly. At this time, the composition of the sweat changes, too, and when it mixes with the bacteria present on the skin, the odor can heighten.

Once you or your child notices an odor, it's definitely time to use deodorant. Some kids feel especially self-conscious about this. Try to be as straightforward and matter-of-fact as possible when you talk to them. Everybody sweats, and it's nothing to be embarrassed about. Here are a few other tips you may find helpful:

- Encourage your child to shower daily, use an antibacterial soap, and gently scrub under their arms and in their groin (where the pubic area meets the legs). Girls should never insert soap into the vaginal canal because it can cause irritation.

- Wash clothes regularly. This is not a time to rewear that T-shirt from gym class. If your child was sweating into their clothes, chances are, the clothes smell.

- Wear breathable fabrics. Cotton breathes much better than spandex, which can trap the odor and magnify the smell. When your child exercises, it's best to wear materials that won't harbor an odor.

:• Encourage your child to stay hydrated. Some evidence suggests that drinking at least eight glasses of water a day keeps the body smelling better. For this and other health-related reasons, proper hydration is very important.

Sometimes you may not notice that your child smells bad because you are just used to their body and all of its emanations. Or perhaps you aren't with your child all day when they are sweaty and emitting a great deal of body odor. As a sexuality educator tackling puberty with young people, Logan is often charged with talking to students about the importance of deodorant. She has worked with many teachers who say that their classrooms stink. (And sometimes they do!)

Some parents don't want to tackle this issue. You may feel like your child is too young for deodorant or that they don't really need it. As someone with one foot in the home and the other in the classroom, Logan offers the following advice: if your child is talking about his or her classmates using deodorant and doesn't use deodorant yet, let her go with you to the drugstore to pick something out. It's time. If your child's teacher is telling you at a conference that your child needs to work on his hygiene, you are being told (albeit nicely) that your kid needs deodorant.

But this doesn't have to be embarrassing. Ideally, all of us use deodorant. And no one really wants to smell bad. It's a milestone, the first deodorant. And there are so many different types and scents available that your kid doesn't have to smell like Old Spice. Deodorant is a very personal choice. Give your child the freedom to choose; it is a small but significant act of ownership for them.

7 This sucks for everyone in our house. When will it end?

Puberty happens at a different pace for everyone, so it's important not to pay close attention to what's going on around you. Everyone catches up. Your son and his best friend might have been born days apart yet could start and end puberty years apart—it's totally normal. Although there are statistics and averages pertaining to when puberty starts and ends, it's really hard to predict; the time frame varies from person to person.

To us, there is nothing worse than hearing a parent tell their kid, "Puberty sucks, but everyone has to go through it." Puberty can be challenging, but how are our kids supposed to feel good about their bodies when we support their claims that these experiences suck? Menstruating doesn't suck; having a wet dream doesn't suck. (Okay, yes, pimples suck. That's different.)

But with respect to the whole "suckage" question: The first thing we would do is reframe this conversation. "Honey, I know that this seems overwhelming, but puberty really is an amazing time in your life. I get that it's confusing and you feel out of sorts, but it happens for a good reason, and I'm here to help make this easier for you. Puberty is a process that takes years, and every person goes through it at their own pace."

Sure, you can acknowledge that there is an "end" to it, but we don't know when that is. So, instead of focusing on that, encourage your child to concentrate on what would make this transitional time more manageable for him or her. Your attitude as a parent can go a long way in influencing your child's take on this whole puberty thing.

PART 2:
IS MY LITTLE BOY BECOMING A MAN?

HERE'S A QUICK look at the stages of puberty for a boy. While the process involves specific ages and stages, based on statistics and national averages, it's important to keep in mind that every boy matures at a different rate. He may go through the stages in order, but he may not. It can be unsettling for your child if his best friend has a growth spurt before he does, or if he is the first to grow facial hair in the class. For parents, it can be equally nerveracking worrying about whether their child has reached puberty too early or too late. Keep in mind that there is a wide range of normal, and encourage your son not to pay too close attention to what's happening to his friends. They will all catch up eventually.

On average, boys begin puberty by the age of eleven or twelve and usually complete the process by age sixteen or seventeen.

According to a 2012 study by the American Academy of Pediatrics (AAP), boys in the United States are reaching puberty roughly six months to two years earlier than a few decades ago, reflecting a similar trend in girls. The same study revealed that African American boys are more likely to enter puberty earlier than white or Hispanic boys. More studies are needed to fully understand the underlying factors responsible for these national trends, but researchers point to a number of possibilities, including nutrition, increased weight and fat distribution, and exposure to environmental toxins and hormonal disruptors.

THE TANNER STAGES OF PUBERTY IN BOYS

The Tanner scale is a scale that health professionals use to measure physical changes in the development of children, teenagers, and adults. These changes vary tremendously, as different people develop at different rates.

- **Stage 1:** The prepubertal stage (immediately before puberty), wherein children usually experience a period of accelerated growth.

- **Stage 2:** Increase in the size of the testicles and scrotal sac; the sac gets darker in color and coarser in texture. Beginning stages of pubic-hair growth: sparse growth, a little bit darker in color, usually at the base of the penis.

- **Stage 3**: Lengthening of the penis and further growth of the testes. Darker, coarser, and curlier hair that spreads over the pubic region.

- **Stage 4**: Penis continues to grow fuller; testes and scrotal sac continue to enlarge and darken in color. Pubic hair continues to fill in.

- **Stage 5**: Adult genitalia are formed; full pubic hair distribution.

Boys also experience the deepening of their voice, the growth of facial and underarm hair, and acne. Puberty that starts earlier than normal is known as precocious puberty. Puberty that starts later than usual is known as delayed puberty.

1 My son is upset because his friends are shaving but he isn't. What should I tell him?

If you put a boy next to a man, one of the most dramatic differences you'll often notice is the amount of hair the man has. Hair growth is one of the major changes your son will experience during puberty. On average, hair growth occurs in specific phases, but bear in mind that this, too, can vary tremendously from person to person.

Here's what you can expect:

∴ Hair grows on the face. It usually starts with a soft, thin mustache on the upper lip that thickens over time.

∴ Hair starts to grow on his cheeks, chin, and neck.

∴ Underarm hair grows next and follows a pattern similar to that of facial hair. It starts out soft and thin at first and gets darker and thicker over time.

∴ The hair on the arms and legs starts to darken and can get thicker as well. This change may be more noticeable in some boys and less in others.

∴ Toward the end of puberty (usually later in the teen years), some boys grow hair on the chest, back, and rear end.

Most boys who have dark hair on their heads usually have dark body hair that tends to be more visible. Boys with lighter hair colors may have very light body hair, but they may not. It is not uncommon for blond-headed boys to have darker underarm or pubic hair. Some boys even have darker facial hair. This is nothing to be concerned about.

Your son may be totally psyched about these new changes, or he may not be enthusiastic at all. He may also want to shave. There are tons of products available for shaving, but remind your son that once he starts, keeping up with hair growth can be a high-maintenance commitment.

Shaving is often a sensitive subject. Even if your son is committed to shaving, you may feel differently about it. Here's the thing: shaving is one of those rites of passage, and in a perfect world, one that's done with some parental supervision, so pick your battles. If this is an important one, that's cool; if it's not, let it go. What's better is to talk about how to shave safely and to explain why shaving is a, dare we say, lifelong commitment, once your child starts.

2 My son was Googling information about penis development. I'm worried he thinks his penis isn't normal.

It is not uncommon for a boy going through puberty—and his parents, for that matter—to wonder or worry about the development and growth of his penis. Doctors treating pubertal males are often asked about the average length of a teenager's penis. While the growth rate varies from person to person, most boys will notice a change between ages ten and fourteen, and it usually occurs after pubic hair appears. Some boys will reach full penile growth very early (age thirteen or fourteen), while others may not experience full growth until well into their late teens. The penis stops growing once puberty ends; many boys' genitalia are close to their adult size by age sixteen.

The penis has several parts:

:• **The shaft**: the main, long part of the penis

:• **The glans**: the tip or head of the penis

:• **The foreskin**: skin that covers the glans (in some boys, this skin is removed for religious, cultural, or health-related reasons)

Underneath the penis is the scrotum—a sac composed of loose, wrinkly skin that hangs down behind a boy's penis, containing the testicles (aka testes or balls). The testicles have two primary functions: to produce testosterone (the male hormone responsible for many of the changes that occur during puberty) and to manufacture and store sperm. It is not uncommon for one of the testicles to hang lower than the other.

In every class Logan has ever taught, she has been asked, "How big is the world's biggest penis?" To which she responds, "I have no idea, and, more importantly, it doesn't really matter. Because really, when you think about it, does having the biggest penis in the world really matter? And would you want that kind of attention?"

You can imagine how surprised students are to hear that. Like every other question they ask, this one falls under the umbrella of "Am I normal?" We need to reassure our sons that there is no one right penis size and that during adolescence their body and their penis are growing. This will save you and your child a great deal of locker-room anxiety.

3 **My son has already experienced a few changes, but he doesn't have any pubic hair yet. Is that normal?**

Not to worry—there's such a wide range of normalcy when it comes to this process. Puberty doesn't start at the same time for everyone, and it doesn't progress in the same way all the time, either. For some children, the stages are predictable; for others, it's more of a crapshoot. Some boys notice a size increase in their genital region but grow very little hair, while others become very hairy but still have high voices. So many factors—including genes, the environment, and nutrition—determine when your son's body undergoes all of the changes puberty has in store for him.

Pubic hair often starts off thin, soft, and light in color. It usually shows up first at the base of the penis. As your son progresses through puberty, the hair turns darker, curlier, and coarser in texture. In boys, it often spreads in a diamond-shaped pattern through the genital region. Over the next few years, the hair will cover the pubic region and can spread out toward the thighs. In general, approximately two years after pubic hair shows up, facial hair, underarm, and chest hair will develop. But remember, these patterns can vary from person to person, too.

4 My girlfriend confused my son for my daughter on the phone last week. He was mortified. When will his voice change?

While being mistaken for a girl may be frustrating for your son (though, we have to say, this is probably a good time to mention that there is nothing wrong with being mistaken for a girl), it is often impossible to tell a boy from a girl over the phone before puberty is complete.

Voice changes and deepening are one of the many changes your son will experience during puberty. Both boys and girls go through these changes, but in girls, they're usually less noticeable. And it doesn't happen overnight. You may notice his voice get squeaky but then return to baseline. It's a process, and the length of time it takes to reach its final depth and pitch varies from person to person.

Our voice comes from our vocal cords, located in the larynx, or voice box. Voice changes occur because as testosterone gets produced during puberty, it causes the larynx to grow and the cords to thicken and elongate. These changes deepen the voice. For most boys, the process lasts a few months. During the process, your son's voice can produce all sorts of unpredictable noises, from squeaking to cracking. Once the voice box and vocal cords finish growing, his voice will settle into a deeper, more adult-sounding tone.

The voice-change process usually occurs between ages fourteen and sixteen in most boys. But there is a tremendous amount of variation, so your son shouldn't be concerned if he is the only tenor in the company of many baritones. He will most likely catch up to his friends.

But let's say that he doesn't catch up. Let's say that he is one of those young men with a higher voice. Adam Levine, anyone? Yes, the lead singer of Maroon 5 and coach on *The Voice* has a crazy falsetto going on, and he is one of the hottest musicians out there. No one said that having a voice like Barry White's makes you more of a man. We don't make assumptions here.

5 My son mentioned that when some of his friends chug water after practice, a bump moves up and down the front of their necks. His dad has this, too, but he doesn't. Will he get one?

Your son may have noticed a lump in the middle of his throat that grows during puberty. This is known as an Adam's apple, and if he wants to feel it, he can take three fingers and place them on the front portion of his throat. When he starts talking, he will feel something moving up and down and vibrating a little. That's his larynx, or voice box. The voice box and vocal cords are protected by cartilage, called the thyroid cartilage. During puberty, just as your son's larynx grows under the influence of hormones, the cartilage that surrounds it grows, too.

The Adam's apple is usually more prominent in boys. Some boys have larger Adam's apples than other boys, while some have no protrusion at all. All of this is normal and can vary from person to person.

6 Why is my son's best friend as tall as LeBron James, when my son is still so short?

One of the more dramatic and noticeable changes of puberty is a period of rapid growth that usually occurs earlier in girls than boys. That's one of the reasons those middle school dances may feel and look awkward: The girls tend to tower over the boys. But the boys will catch up. According to statistics from the American Academy of Pediatrics, the average boy experiences a growth spurt around age thirteen and a half, roughly two years later than the average girl.

The growth rate during adolescence is the fastest your child will ever experience, aside from when he was a baby. And it's not just your son's height that will increase; his hands, arms, legs, and feet will grow quickly and sometimes cause temporary clumsiness before the rest of his body catches up. As his trunk lengthens, his thighs will get wider and his shoulders will broaden. Even the facial bones will grow, and in some boys, a squaring of the jaw is noticeable—which can change the appearance of their face.

But, as with everything else in puberty, the rate of height and weight changes can vary. Some boys may grow several inches in a month and stop, and then grow some more, while others experience a more gradual course that they don't really notice until their yearly doctor's appointment when they are told they've shot up five inches.

Your son shouldn't be concerned if he is the shortest in his class in the fall; all of that can easily change by the spring. In addition, there can be considerable variation within a family; brothers and sisters may grow at different rates.

That being said, if you happen to have a child who is on the smaller side (even for the time being), it can make him feel very insecure socially. At a time when our young people are starting to develop crushes, date, kiss, and so on, "small" boys sometimes feel left out because they may be perceived as more "boy" and less "teen." So be supportive and let your son know that we all develop at our own pace.

Parents also need to encourage healthy lifestyle habits during this time, because all of this growth can be exhausting for your child, who needs the proper amount of rest and good nutrition. This is not a time to diet. Top priorities should include the following:

- **Sleep:** Because the body is working overtime growing in all directions, your child needs his rest. Doctors recommend ten to twelve hours of uninterrupted sleep every night.

:• **Good nutrition:** This is vital for lowering the risk of obesity, a problem that can interfere with hormone production and proper growth patterns.

:• **Regular exercise:** Many experts recommend twenty to thirty minutes of exercise per day for kids, which can help strengthen growing muscles and bones, reduce the risk of obesity, and lower the levels of stress hormones in the body.

7 While changing in the locker room, my son noticed his friend's uncircumcised penis and is asking some questions that I'm not sure how to answer.

Not all penises are the same. This is a good lesson, because puberty is a time when our sons are trying to "measure up" to others. And, as we know, the penis, though it's just a body part, is a source of great pride and sometimes great stress. While they may not necessarily admit it, boys do surreptitiously check each other out in the locker rooms or at sleepover dates because they want to know if their penis is "normal." (Now, you know how we feel about that word already: There's no such thing as normal.)

We like to say that penises come in two varieties: circumcised and uncircumcised. One is not better than the other (though there has been much debate about health benefits and sensitivity in recent years). Circumcision is a personal—and, quite frankly, a parental—choice.

The foreskin, also known medically as the prepuce, is a loose fold of skin that covers the head of the penis. Although the rates have declined slightly in recent years, the majority of American men were circumcised at birth or as infants; the exact percentage varies depending on the source. However, the majority of men worldwide have uncircumcised penises.

The benefits of circumcision have been called into question in the new millennium, but after a comprehensive review of scientific evidence, the American Academy of Pediatrics found that the health benefits of newborn male circumcision outweigh the risks. Still, the AAP stopped short of recommending universal newborn circumcision, because it found that the benefits are not great enough to do so. The World Health Organization (WHO) endorsed male circumcision as "an important intervention to reduce the risk of heterosexually acquired HIV."

Many parents in the United States decide to circumcise their sons for religious or aesthetic reasons. Parents we have spoken to said that they wanted their sons to look like their fathers. There are also some hygiene issues with uncircumcised penises. The foreskin doesn't retract easily at first, but by the time your son is five, the foreskin should be fully retractable. At this point, cleaning under the foreskin is important, to get rid of smegma, a thick, white secretion made up of dead skin cells and natural lubricating residue. Girls can get this, too; it tends to build up around the clitoris and labia minora. By the time puberty hits, boys should be instructed to clean under the foreskin regularly. Also important to note is that if the foreskin doesn't retract fully by the time your son reaches puberty, you need to call your doctor for advice. You should never forcibly retract the foreskin.

8 Do all boys wake up with erections? And if this happens to my son in class, what should he do?

Boys have been capable of having an erection since they were little—in fact, male fetuses can get erections in utero—but during puberty, they get erections frequently and unexpectedly, without stimulating themselves or having sexual thoughts of any kind. It's not uncommon for these erections to occur at the most unwanted and inconvenient moments, like when a boy is giving a presentation in class or thinking about how much he *doesn't* want an erection.

Involuntary erections can definitely be embarrassing but are a normal part of puberty and body development. Many boys feel better knowing that this has happened to every other boy they know, and that it becomes less and less frequent as they get older.

Logan loves to talk about erections in class, because there is nothing better than seeing a boy's face when he figures out that his erections are part of natural development, rather than something that is wrong with his body.

Compare erections to a sponge. When a sponge fills with water, it expands. When the spongy-tissue inside of the penis fills with blood, it expands in the same way. Logan has found that once boys understand that their erections are normal, they become more concerned with practical issues, such as the following:

Question: What if I get an erection in school?

Answer: You will, and it may be embarrassing, so if you're walking down the hallway when it happens, just casually carry a notebook or book in front of your pants. If you don't touch your erection and try not to worry about it, it will go away.

Question: How am I supposed to pee when I have an erection?

Answer: You're right—that's not easy. You're probably going to have to wait a few minutes for it to go away. If you don't, you're going to wind up spraying pee all over the bathroom—and you're going to have to clean it up. (And we know that's the last thing you want to do.)

Question: Why did I get an erection when I saw someone/something that I don't like?

Answer: For no reason at all. You can't always control when you have an erection. You can get one if you're nervous or uncomfortable, if someone accidentally brushes up against you, if you see someone you like, if you see someone you don't like. It doesn't necessarily mean anything.

In the end, consider all of these topics part of erection management. A boy can't stop himself from getting an erection, but he can shorten the amount of time that he has one. Or, as we all know, he can extend that time—but we've tackled masturbation already.

9 I've noticed some wet, sticky spots on my son's sheets in the morning lately. He seems embarrassed. Should I discuss this with him?

Most boys will experience the sensation of waking up with wet pajamas or wet sheets/blankets at some point during puberty. It's all normal and nothing to be ashamed of. As we mentioned, erections can occur at any time, even at night. When the erection is accompanied by an ejaculation—known as a nocturnal emission, or "wet dream"—your son may wake up in the middle of the night, worried that he's wet his bed. But if he's going through puberty, the chances are much higher that he's had a wet dream.

When boys go through puberty, their bodies start to produce the male hormone testosterone. As testosterone circulates in the body, sperm gains the potential to be released. A wet dream is when semen, the fluid that contains sperm, gets expelled from the penis during sleep. It's important to note that with the ability to release sperm comes along the ability to get a girl pregnant through vaginal intercourse.

Some boys worry that something is wrong with them, but nothing could be further from the truth. Wet dreams are a normal part of puberty, and their frequency subsides over time. Other boys worry that they *aren't* having wet dreams. Although they are common, not every teenage boy will experience them, and that's normal, too.

But consider how complicated the nocturnal emission really is. On the one hand, wet dreams seem fairly grown-up; on the other hand, they remind boys of peeing in their beds. It's challenging for them to separate urine from semen at this point, because they probably haven't ever ejaculated and haven't seen semen or any other ejaculatory fluid before.

There's another component to wet-dream anxiety that we'd be remiss not to bring up: cleaning the sheets. More specifically, boys are often afraid that you'll say something to them or be upset by what they have done. Logan has explained time and time again to her students that any parent or caregiver of a near-adolescent male understands that wet dreams are part of sexual development, but the subject still makes them uncomfortable. As parents, we need to tell boys that we won't ask questions or be upset by this event—it's just part of life.

🔟 My son's chest seems to be developing a little. WTF?

Think about one of the most noticeable (and often very exciting) parts of female puberty for boys: breast development. And no, we're not suggesting that all of our sons are heterosexual. We're merely stating that breasts are the first obviously physical image of what separates the males from the females. And while your son may not be into girls romantically, breasts can be fascinating— especially because they're not on his body.

Now imagine being a boy and having your own (small for female but big for male) breasts. It can be completely embarrassing. Even though the development of breast tissue is a normal part of puberty for many boys, it's not the easiest topic to address. Reactions can range from embarrassment to denial to horror. No matter what the response is, it's important to recognize that the majority of boys going through puberty are going to experience some breast growth. These changes are caused by hormones that act to develop secondary sex characteristics in boys. Some of the hormones originate from female hormones, and as the levels get higher, breast development can occur temporarily.

Here's what you can expect: During the earlier parts of puberty, most boys will experience some swelling, discomfort, or tenderness around their nipples. According to the American Academy of Pediatrics, actual breast growth will occur in at least 75 percent of boys, or three in four. Some boys will notice it, some will not. Most of the time, the growth is confined to the nipple area; in other cases, the growth is more pronounced. Some boys notice that the skin around the nipple (areola) gets darker and wider. The nipples may become slightly larger, too.

Let's get the bad news out of the way: There's no way around this. Adolescent boys are quite sensitive to being ridiculed, and breast growth is certainly a potential source of public embarrassment. In the warmer months, you can encourage your son to wear a T-shirt or loose-fitting rash guard with his bathing suits.

The good news is, breast growth usually *does* go away, typically within one to two years. If it doesn't, a trip to the doctor may be necessary. There are several medical conditions that cause excessive breast growth in boys and men, including thyroid disease, chromosomal disorders, and tumors of the endocrine system. Breast growth in boys and men can also be a side effect of certain medications or the result of being overweight or obese. All of these conditions are best addressed by a medical professional.

Sometimes we find it helpful to explicitly state that both boys and girls have breasts. For some reason, we feel like that word—*breasts*—is owned by girls. That is what makes this issue so challenging for boys. They can't imagine breast growth being normal, because "boys aren't supposed to have breasts." It's just not that simple.

11 **All my son's friends look much more built than he is, and he's concerned. Does he need to work out 24-7 to get big muscles?**

Body image isn't just an issue for females. Boys, too, get their own dose of insecurities from mass media and pop culture telling them to be big, have washboard abs, be strong, be a man. Not every male was meant to look this way; not every person is attracted to this look, contrary to what we watch on television or in films. Set the stage by explaining this early, and then follow up with the facts.

Just as some boys will grow taller more rapidly than others, some will develop muscles and increase muscle mass faster than others. Puberty is not a race, but it's natural to feel insecure if those around you are bulking up and you're not. For many boys, an increase in muscle mass accompanies a growth spurt. Your son will grow a few inches, his shoulders will become broader, and his weight will increase as his muscle mass grows.

It's not uncommon for boys to be concerned about their muscles. Even if they are experiencing some of the changes of puberty, muscle growth doesn't happen overnight—they won't go to sleep one day and wake up looking like a bodybuilder in the morning. Sometimes certain muscle groups develop before others. For example, the deltoid (shoulder) muscles could develop before the pectoralis (chest) muscles, leaving boys feeling a bit lopsided. This imbalance usually lasts only a short time, until the body catches up. Everyone is different and develops at his own pace.

If your son decides that he wants to work out and lift weights, consult a doctor or medical professional who can point him in the right direction. To avoid injury and avoid overdoing it, he should start off by speaking with a qualified coach or trainer who can recommend the proper amount of weight for him to lift (which can vary significantly from person to person) and identify how much time his body needs to recover between sessions.

Finally, remember that your son should be taking care of himself and his body because he wants to, not because he thinks others will like or accept him more.

PART 3:
IS MY LITTLE GIRL BECOMING A WOMAN?

H ERE'S A QUICK look at the stages of puberty for a girl. While the process involves specific ages and stages, based on statistics and national averages, it's important to keep in mind that every girl matures at different rates. She may go through the stages in order, but she may not. It can be unsettling for your child if she gets her period before her best friend or if she is the last to develop breasts in her class. For parents, it can be equally nerve-racking worrying about whether their child has reached puberty too early or too late. Just ask parents who have chaperoned a seventh-grade dance or attended an eighth-grade recital: Some girls are fully developed, while others haven't grown an inch since fifth grade. Keep in mind that there is a wide range of normal, and encourage your daughter not to pay too close attention to what's happening to her friends. They will all catch up eventually.

On average, girls begin puberty by the age of ten or eleven and usually complete the process by age fifteen to seventeen. Several studies have shown that girls are entering puberty at earlier ages than they have in the past. A study in the journal *Pediatrics* revealed that African American and Hispanic girls mature faster than Caucasian girls. Roughly 25 percent of African American girls and 15 percent of Hispanic girls had entered puberty by the age of seven, according to this study. Experts weren't sure of the exact cause, but a combination of factors—including the childhood obesity epidemic and substances in the environment—is likely.

The Tanner scale of puberty for girls describes only breast and pubic hair development and does *not* include vaginal growth. In most girls, the vagina grows longer and its outer and inner lips (labia majora and minora, respectively) become more pronounced over the course of several years, usually between the ages of eight and fifteen. Menstruation is also not part of this system, but a girl's first menstrual period can occur at Tanner stage 2, 3, 4, or even 5. On average, girls in the United States experience their first period between ages twelve and thirteen, across all cultural and ethnic groups.

THE TANNER STAGES OF PUBERTY IN GIRLS

:• **Stage 1:** Preadolescent breasts.

:• **Stage 2**: Breast tissue starts to develop with the onset of areola (a darker circle around each nipple) enlargement, often forming a separate mound. Sparse, straight, and soft labial pubic hair develops.

:• **Stage 3**: Breasts grow in size and assume a more rounded contour. Pubic hair becomes darker, coarser, and curlier and starts to extend laterally.

:• **Stage 4**: Increased breast size and elevation, growing closer to adult shape. Pubic hair distribution broadens across pubic area.

:• **Stage 5**: Breasts reach mature adult shape and size. Adult pubic hair distribution extends to include the medial thighs.

① Which will my daughter get first: breasts, her period, or hair under her arms?

The answer to this question depends on many different factors, and the stages can vary significantly between your daughter and her friends. So let's start by explaining what is going on in her body and when she can expect these changes to occur. The first thing that happens is something she won't be able to see if she looks in the mirror. The pituitary gland (an endocrine gland about the size

of a pea), which is located at the base of the brain, releases a chemi-
cal signal that tells your daughter's ovaries (reproductive organs
found in her pelvis) to start producing the female sex hormone,
estrogen. Circulating estrogen will then trigger the maturation process of the reproductive organs—the ovaries, uterus, and fallopian
tubes—so her body will be prepared to bear children sometime in
the future. Estrogen also causes the development of secondary sex
characteristics in girls, which include breast formation, broadening
of the hips, and fat redistribution. These and other changes occur
over a number of years.

For many girls, one of the first signs of puberty is the development of breast buds, which on average begins at some point between
the ages of eight and thirteen. It usually starts with a bit of swelling
under one or both nipples, developing into a nickel-size lump/bud;
girls often report feelings of soreness and tenderness, too. Some girls
have difficulty sleeping on their stomachs during this stage. It is also
not uncommon for one breast to develop before the other; actually,
in roughly 50 percent of American adult women, one breast tends
to be larger than the other. The difference is usually so slight that
no one notices, and there's no cause for concern.

The next change for many girls is the growth of pubic hair. The
hair usually starts off soft, thin, and light in color, growing straight
on the outer labia, then darkens, thickens, becomes curlier, and
spreads out as girls move through puberty. Pubic hair generally
begins to appear after breasts start to develop but may appear first
in some girls; this is all normal.

On average, roughly two years after your daughter's breasts start to develop, she may get her first period. It may come and go in the beginning and not stick to a regular schedule. It will get on track over time. Again, some girls get their period earlier or later than others, or out of order within all of these stages. Underarm hair tends to grow in a little later, between the ages of eleven and sixteen for many girls. It's important to realize that all of these changes can vary tremendously from person to person. Puberty is an individual sport, and every girl's experience is different. There's a wide range of normal, so your daughter shouldn't freak out if her experience is different from her sister's or her best friend's.

❷ Why is my daughter getting breasts before any of her friends? She feels embarrassed and asked me if it's because she's fat.

In a world dominated by competing images of adult film stars and emaciated actresses, it is easy to imagine why your daughter is consumed with insecurities about how she looks.

For a young girl, breast development is akin to a giant, flashing neon arrow pointing to her chest: LOOK HERE. BREASTS HERE. CHECK 'EM OUT. Sure, that's definitely not how your daughter is feeling; she's probably trying to do anything to *avoid* drawing attention to her developing breasts, but that's almost impossible, especially if she is one of the first in her class to show signs of development.

Add to that the messed-up representations of bodies we see in pop culture, and it shouldn't surprise us that our girls are anxious about being perceived as "fat." So you have to think carefully about where this question is coming from. Your daughter is really asking two questions: 1) *Why am I the first to get breasts?* 2) *Am I fat?*

As with many questions, this question may have to do with whether your daughter is "normal," but what she really wants to know is how to manage these developments that are happening in her before her friends and peers experience them. This conversation is a nuanced one, and you're going to need to tackle her questions one at a time. Breast development occurs first, weight and body image second.

So here goes: The medical term for early puberty is *precocious puberty*, which is when someone experiences puberty a little earlier than the average age range for puberty onset. If the process starts before the age of seven or eight in a girl or age nine in a boy, it meets the clinical criteria for precocious puberty.

Precocious puberty is more common in girls than in boys, in kids who are overweight or obese, and it can be inherited. The signs of precocious puberty are the same as the signs for puberty, and, like puberty, the entire process can take two and a half to three years.

As with regular-onset puberty, one of the first indications of puberty in a girl is usually the development of her breasts, which begins with a small, often tender mound underneath the nipples. The breasts can develop asymmetrically; this is completely normal.

Breast development is usually followed by the growth of pubic hair, some body odor, and possibly acne, because the sweat and oil glands become more active in the body during this time. As these changes occur, your daughter may experience vaginal discharge and hormone-related mood swings, and eventually she will start menstruating. Underarm hair growth is often one of the last changes of puberty. On average, the entire process takes two and a half to three years but can take longer in some girls. Being overweight or obese can trigger puberty-related changes earlier than normal.

At the heart of parents' and children's concerns during this period is whether children are "normal." First and foremost, it's worth mentioning to your daughter that the signs of puberty vary tremendously from person to person, and that she may experience these changes in a different order than her friends undergo them.

It's also very important to note that rapid weight gain for girls is a natural part of the process. In fact, it would be unhealthy if your daughter didn't gain weight during this time. On average, most girls can expect to gain between fifteen and twenty pounds during puberty.

As for the embarrassment factor, children of any age often feel embarrassed as they experience puberty, because these very personal changes are very public. Many pubescent developments are visible to others; in fact, other people sometimes notice these changes before children themselves do. (Imagine how vulnerable you would feel if someone commented that they saw little breast buds peeking out of your T-shirt.) Even parents' physical responses to their children during this time seem to change, too. When our daughters develop breasts, sometimes we shy away from hugging them (especially fathers), because, mentally, we feel like the breasts get in the way.

Puberty is the first real time in young people's lives when they notice their bodies, not just their faces. This experience can be even more difficult for younger girls, who don't have the emotional maturity to handle these changes. In addition, girls who struggle with their weight during childhood may face additional body-image issues that precocious puberty only compounds. If you think your daughter is having a hard time in this regard, a health care professional can help determine if there is an underlying issue, and whether and how to manage excess weight gain. Doctors often keep track of height and weight changes during childhood, so they can chart out your daughter's growth during puberty and help figure out an optimal plan for her.

If you have a child who is struggling with body image as it relates to her new, pubescent body, remind her that her body is beautiful. Tell her that you understand how hard it is to feel like a child but have a more grown-up body. Let her know that what she is experiencing is something that everyone goes through, just not at the same time. Sometimes it's hard to be the first, but people will catch up. (Sometimes it's hard to be the last, too.) And whatever you and your parenting partner (if you have one) do, don't stop hugging your daughters. Make sure that they know that you still love them, regardless of their breasts.

③ My daughter just asked if she could have a push-up bra. Yikes!

One thing is certain: Developing girls today have more bra options than ever before. The days of the old training bra are over. Today, in addition to all of the traditional styles, girls can wear sports bras, bikini-looking bras, and tank tops with built-in bras.

When Logan was young, it was painfully obvious that she was the first girl in her class to wear a bra. The straps were far from inconspicuous, and the boys loved to snap them. Girls who want to quietly manage their breast development have many more opportunities to do so now than in the past. And these intermediary bras, or bralettes, are super comfortable. Truth be told, Logan would still much rather wear those.

Now, don't get us wrong—we are not suggesting that all girls are uncomfortable with their breast development, nor do we think they should be. However, there is a difference between the desire to wear a bra (or to have actual breasts) and wanting to push them up. We have trolled the aisles of many clothing stores and are quite horrified by the concept of push-up bras for young girls. For us, this has to do with the insidious (and sometimes overt) sexualization of girls. To look "sexy," before you even know what sexy is (or feel it), is unhealthy. Girls need to be learning to love their bodies. Push-up bras say, *Look at my breasts!* or, *The only way to be pretty is to prop those puppies up—even when you hardly have them.*

If your daughter comes to you wanting a push-up bra, please understand that she is simply asking because that's what our culture has told her is beautiful and sexy, and even though she may not understand what that means, she does know that our world recognizes beauty and sex appeal as serious commodities. In the end, the decision is yours, but we encourage you to consider the following issues and explain them to your daughter:

:• As fate has it, youthful breasts are already pushed up. That's one of the benefits of being younger.

:• Your body is beautiful as it is. You haven't even finished developing yet, and you already want to make changes to it? There's no need for that.

Now, we know what you're thinking: *Didn't either of you ever stuff your bra or try to make your breasts bigger?* Actually, no. If you read this book's introduction, you know all about Logan's "soccer ball tits." If not, consider the difference: Stuffing one's bra to have the appearance of breasts (when you don't have any yet and your peers do) is very different from pushing those already-perky breasts up to the sky so that other people can look at them.

In the end, you're the parent; it's your decision. But we do feel like it's our responsibility to encourage our children to feel good about themselves, not to give them products that perpetuate the idea that they are inadequate.

4 **My daughter is freaked out by the prospect of getting her period. She thinks it's totally gross.**

Please. Please. We need to help our daughters change their perspective by rephrasing what is going happening during puberty. Can we avoid using the term *gross* when we speak about menstruation? It may seem messy, but the body is actually amazing. And while the process can be overwhelming, scary, or mysterious for some girls, understanding why it happens is crucial. Because of a girl's period, her body will be able to create and bring life into this world, if—yes, *if*—she so chooses, at some point in the future.

Menstruation is part of the reproductive cycle. Every month, one of your daughter's ovaries will release an egg. This process is called ovulation. The egg makes its way through the fallopian tubes into the uterus. Hormones in the body trigger changes in the uterus, thickening its lining to prepare the body for pregnancy. If the egg released during ovulation isn't fertilized by sperm from a male (this can happen only through vaginal intercourse, in vitro fertilization, or artificial insemination), it starts to break down and passes out of the body, along with the built-up lining of the uterus that dissolves without a fertilized egg. This cycle is called a period.

There is quite a bit of variation in menstruation, but the average period occurs every twenty-eight to thirty days and lasts roughly four to six days. The amount of blood the female's body loses in the process can vary quite a bit, too. It may seem like a lot, but, on average, most girls lose much less blood than they think.

On average, menstruating girls change their pads about three to five times a day. The first two days of their period tend to produce heavier blood flow, which usually tapers off toward the middle to end of the cycle.

Having a period is an extraordinary experience, though we know it's not always convenient. Logan had her period at her senior prom, at her wedding, and during her honeymoon. Jena got her period just as the pilot turned off the seat belt sign on her way to her honeymoon. But we need to stop suggesting to our girls (and our boys) that periods are a necessary evil. How on earth can they embrace their bodies (or others') if they perceive themselves as gross? It's not a curse; it is blessing and a power that half of the world's population doesn't have. All of us need to do a better job at reframing the issue of menstruation as a positive, not a negative.

5 My daughter got her period once but hasn't had it for a few months. Could she be pregnant?

Girls going through puberty have probably been told at some point that menstruation is a predictable cycle and that they will get their period once a month. But keep in mind that a pubertal girl's body may not follow a tight schedule, especially in the first one to two years after she first gets her period. It is not uncommon for girls to have an irregular menstrual cycle or even to even skip their period for several months at a time.

It's also common for the levels of menstruation-related hormones to vary from one cycle to the next and thereby cause the amount of blood and the duration of the period to vary as well. Sometimes a period lasts a week; other times it lasts only a few days. All of this is normal and usually evens out as a girl gets older. Many young women will report experiencing a regular pattern up to roughly three years after their first period.

Some girls develop irregular periods or stop having them altogether because of different factors that a medical professional may need to address. These can include stress, rapid weight loss, excessive exercise, illness, some medications, and imbalances of female sex hormones. Disorders of the thyroid gland can cause irregular periods, as can polycystic ovary syndrome, which can cause the female body to produce excess androgen, a male hormone that results in menstrual irregularities, deepening of the voice, facial hair, and weight gain.

All these possibilities aside, if a girl is sexually active and has missed a period, it could be a sign that she is pregnant. She may want to take a pregnancy test; most tests will provide a reliable result one week after a missed period. If the test is positive, it is important for your daughter to speak to someone she trusts and make an appointment with a health care provider who can best guide her.

6 **My daughter is sleeping over at her friend's house and will have her period while she's there. She doesn't know whether she should tell her friend. I'm not sure how to advise her on this.**

On the first day of sixth grade, Logan drew a giant dot on her best friend's notebook page. "Logan, what is that?" the friend asked. She drew it again. And again. And again. Five seconds later, there were hundreds of dots all over the page but the friend still couldn't figure out what Logan was cryptically trying to tell her. Finally, Logan said, "Periods. Those are periods. I have my period."

"Oh. Okay. Why didn't you just say that?" the friend asked. Lesson learned.

We get pretty wrapped up with right or wrong when it comes to period etiquette, but menstruation is nothing to feel embarrassed by or ashamed of. It's a natural part of puberty that every girl will eventually experience. If your daughter feels comfortable telling her friend, then it's okay to let her know. If she wants to keep it to herself, that's okay, too. It's all up to her, but you may want to ask your daughter if you can tell her friend's mother, just in case she needs a tampon or pad while she is at their house. If your daughter decides she doesn't want anyone to know, make sure she takes some sealable plastic bags with her so that she can dispose of used sanitary products at home.

Also, remind your daughter that she should never flush pads or tampons down a toilet unless she wants to let her friend's whole family in on her little secret. One of Jena's best friends flushed a pad down the toilet at a slumber party and backed up the birthday girl's entire septic system. When the plumber came in the next day, he discovered the extralong pad blocking one of the pipes. After the mom questioned seven girls, Jena's friend who had her period was mortified and turned beet red, so they all knew she was the culprit. That probably wasn't the way that she wanted everyone to find out. So it's wise to instruct your daughter about how to properly dispose of these products.

It's also important to remind her that she may experience certain physical or emotional symptoms when she gets her period that could affect the sleepover.

PHYSICAL SYMPTOMS MAY INCLUDE:

- Cramps
- Fatigue/exhaustion
- Bloating
- Nausea
- Diarrhea or constipation
- Headaches
- Tender, sore breasts
- Change in appetite
- Acne breakouts

EMOTIONAL SYMPTOMS MAY INCLUDE:

- Mood swings
- Sadness or feelings of wanting to cry

:• Difficulty concentrating

:• Frustration or anger

:• Nervous energy or anxiety

:• Disrupted sleep patterns

Some girls experience some of these symptoms with their period; others experience very few to no symptoms. And each period can be different. Our advice: There is no reason for your daughter not to enjoy her sleepover while her body is doing its thing. She should tell her friend only if she feels like it, and be prepared. Women have been menstruating since the beginning of time—there's no need for a menstrual cycle to get in the way of life.

7 My daughter is self-conscious because she is the tallest of all her friends. When will they catch up?

When it comes to growth spurts during puberty, quite a bit of variation occurs. So, just because your daughter is the tallest of all of her friends right now, it doesn't mean this will always be the case. It's important to keep in mind that everyone grows at their own pace.

Can we just repeat that again? *Everyone grows at their own pace.* We desperately want to compare ourselves to others, but we can't—especially during puberty. Logan has been the same height, five foot five, since fourth or fifth grade. She felt like a giant back then, but people caught up, more or less, and she stopped growing. Jena was one of the shortest of all her friends and had a growth spurt a little later than average.

So while your child may feel like a giant or a Smurf, we need to explain that everyone feels the same way at some point. More importantly, we can show our children images of successful people of varying heights in our history or culture. This way, wherever they are height-wise, kids won't associate success with a particular height.

Here are the facts: On average, between ages nine and thirteen, girls experience a growth spurt or a period of time in which they grow much faster than they have grown in the past. The fastest point of growth in girls occurs most commonly at age eleven and a half, roughly two years before the average growth spurt for boys. But then the boys catch up and tend to grow more inches each year than girls do (which is why the average man is taller than the average woman). Most girls stop growing rapidly once they get their period, and gain just a few inches afterward.

Not only do girls grow taller during puberty, but you will notice other changes in your daughter's body shape as well. Girls tend to become curvier during this time, as their hips widen and their breasts develop. Some girls get stretch marks, similar to pregnant women's, because their bodies' rapid growth pulls on their skin. These marks will fade over time.

It is normal for girls to feel confused or uncomfortable about some of the changes that their bodies are going through. Women in our society are conditioned to be aware of their bodies and their weight at very young ages. From a medical perspective, it is not healthy to go on a crash diet to try to stop any pubertal body-shape changes and normal weight gain. As parents, we need to model body appreciation and acceptance for our children. They absorb your message more than you realize, so if you're constantly on a diet or asking out loud if you look fat, your daughter will hear you.

8 My daughter hates the hair growing on her body; she says it's gross. What should I tell her?

There it is again—the *gross* word. As parents, we really need to encourage our children to welcome and accept these changes, not loathe them. Ultimately, we want them to feel good about their bodies and have a strong sense of self-esteem, and we need to model this for them. We can start by reframing the way they speak about puberty.

One of the many changes your child will experience during puberty is the growth of hair in places she was not used to having it before. For girls, hair tends to grow in the pubic area—starting off thin, straight, and soft, later becoming curlier, coarser, and darker, as it spreads out over the entire genital region and sometimes extends to the inner thighs. Hair also grows under the arms, and existing hair on the arms and legs tends to darken and fill in. It's not uncommon for girls to get hair on their faces as well, especially on the upper lip.

During puberty, the adrenal glands react to a signal and begin to produce hormones (androgens) that trigger the growth of hair in both girls and boys. The timing of hair growth tends to follow a pattern but can occur anytime during puberty.

Some girls don't mind the extra hair on their bodies and choose to leave it alone, while others hate it and opt to get rid of it, especially under their arms, on their legs, and on their upper lip. This decision is entirely up to you and your child, but either way you'll definitely want to discuss all the options with your daughter. From shaving to creams, waxing, and bleaching, there are tons of safe products she can use. Just make sure she reads the instructions.

Jena's first experience with hair removal was a disaster. After barely skimming the written insert, she applied globs of the hair-removal cream Nair to her armpits and along her legs. She decided to wait seven minutes. Why seven, you ask? She liked the number. She then jumped into the shower, hoping to scrub away all of her unwanted hair, but when only some of the hair came off, she decided to do what all girls her age would do: apply more cream. Big mistake! Her skin, which was already irritated, became inflamed. Unfortunately, she used the same washcloth to soothe her burning armpits—also not a good idea. At the end of the ordeal, she screamed for her mom, who came to the rescue with cold compresses. Jena opted for shaving after that.

We highly recommend discussing hair removal with someone who knows how to do it successfully. However, no one should feel pressure to get rid of body hair. It's natural in some cultures, trends change all the time, and we need to do what feels right for us, regardless of what (it seems like) everyone else is doing.

9 My daughter just asked for a Brazilian bikini wax for her birthday—hello!

We can't possibly imagine how you'd wrap up a present like that. In case you haven't heard of it before, a Brazilian bikini wax is a grooming technique (and not the most comfortable one) in which the waxer removes all of the pubic hair—from the labia, the anus, the works—and typically leaves a small strip at the top. It was created by, well, Brazilians who wanted no hair showing in their teeny-tiny bikinis. This trend for young people bothers us immensely—not because we don't like Brazilian bikini waxes in general, but because they weren't designed for teenagers who are just starting to have and make sense of their pubic hair.

Grooming pubic hair is a complicated topic. It's easy to encourage young girls not to do it, but if you have ever been a girl with pubic hair coming out of the sides of her bathing suit, you are going to feel very differently. Logan will be the first to admit that she was waxed and "electrolysized" (with her mother's guidance and support) during her youth, but she was taking care of only the hairs on her bikini line, not on her entire genitalia.

Try this on for size: Teenage girls barely through puberty want to take off all their pubic hair before they even know what it is going to look like. And let's not stick our heads in the sand—we propose that if teens are going Brazilian, they aren't the only ones looking at their vulvas. Yes, we said it: Girls (who, in Logan's experience as a sex educator, barely look at genitals and often shout, "Ooh, gross" when she suggests that they do) are not Brazilian waxing for themselves; they are doing it for the other people who will be looking at their vulva.

Girls (and boys, for that matter) need to know that not all women wax it off. Some women prefer to be bushy. In fact, there's an entire Facebook movement dedicated to the appreciation of women's pubic hair, called Bring Back the Bush. There should be no rules about young people's grooming—and that means parents shouldn't have any expectations about it either.

🔟 My daughter's freaking out that her favorite pair of jeans doesn't fit anymore. How should I explain this to her?

As we mentioned before, getting taller isn't the only growth that girls experience during this time; changes in body shape may happen as well. Before puberty, many girls have a more rounded belly, where much of their fat, in the form of adipose (the connective tissue containing fat cells) is stored.

During puberty, the female body experiences a redistribution of fat from the stomach and waist to the breasts, thighs, and hips. In addition, the pelvic bone tends to spread or grow wider and the waist tends to get smaller. Unfortunately, these changes can wreak havoc on your daughter's wardrobe (and your wallet!) by turning her favorite pair of jeans into a hand-me-down overnight.

11 Wait—what is a vulva, anyway?

If your child is asking this, congratulate her for knowing that there is a word *vulva*, and no, she's not referring to a car. What we commonly call the vagina is actually the vulva. The vagina is the passageway inside a girl's body; all of the parts that you can see between a girl's legs—the mons pubis, labis, urethra, vaginal opening, and ever-important clitoris—are all part of the vulva. Vulvas are like flowers. They are all different and yet all beautiful.

What our children should know is what those parts are and what they do. Here's a little review of female anatomy 101 (the external-genitalia edition) for you and your child:

:• **Mons pubis:** The rounded, fatty mass over the pubic bone that is covered with pubic hair. This acts as a buffer during sexual intercourse and prevents injury to the underlying pelvic structures. It contains specialized sweat glands that secrete pheromones (a characteristic odor) that often increase sexual attraction.

:• **Labia majora:** The two outer, rounded folds (outer lips) on either side of the vaginal opening. These form the external, lateral boundary of the vulva. Hair growth over the labia majora is one of the earlier signs of puberty in many girls.

:• **Labia minora:** The inner lips or delicate flaps of soft skin within the labia majora. These fold over and protect the opening of the vagina, urethra, and the clitoris. They come in all different sizes and can vary in shape and texture among different women.

:• **Clitoris:** A bud-like structure that is a highly sensitive erectile organ. This is located near the anterior portion of the vulva, is the primary source of female sexual pleasure, and has legs that extend down the sides of the vulva, behind the labia.

:• **Urethra:** The tube that connects the urinary bladder to the external genitals for the removal of urine from the body.

:• **Vaginal opening:** The exterior opening to the vaginal canal, made of muscle, that extends from the cervix to the outside of the body.

12 **My daughter just asked me if she was dying because there's something wet and disgusting in her underwear.**

It's not disgusting, and she can relax—she's not dying! Girls may begin to notice white or yellow stains inside their underwear during puberty. This substance is called vaginal discharge; it's a fluid that the female body produces and is nature's way of cleaning the vagina, keeping it from becoming too dry, and preventing infections. Big, important point here if you missed it: The vagina cleans itself. It does not need other products to do that. (Take that, douches and any other products marketed to clean the vagina.)

When a girl first notices vaginal discharge, it's typically an indicator that she will get her period in six to eighteen months—though, of course, not everyone follows this time frame.

The amount of discharge can vary throughout the menstrual cycle, as can the consistency. It may or may not have a slight odor; either way is normal. Some girls feel more comfortable wearing panty liners to protect their underwear. Thankfully, if your daughter does want to wear something, she has myriad products to choose from. Many health care professionals recommend choosing unscented products because scented feminine products can cause irritation in some girls and women.

It's important for girls to be aware of any strong odor, change in color, or other symptoms—including redness, soreness, itching, and pain—in their genital area that accompany vaginal discharge. These can all be signs of an infection, so your daughter should seek the assistance of a health care provider who can best treat her, if necessary.

2

Sex Behaviors and Sexual Health

PART 1:
THE INS AND OUTS OF SEX

W E KNOW THAT some of you might prefer to put your head in the sand or talk about just about anything else with your children, but your child needs to discuss this with you more than you may realize. And let's be honest: They're going to learn about it anyway. They will hear things from their friends and older siblings, on television shows and YouTube—you name it. Sex is everywhere, and what they pick up from other sources may be far less accurate than what you can tell them.

An open dialogue with your child about sex and sexuality will ensure that they receive accurate, reliable information, as well as messages consistent with your personal values. Of course, that assumes that you have accurate, reliable information already. If that isn't available to you, keep reading, because conversations between you and your child can help them learn about responsible sexual behavior and acquire healthy attitudes toward sex.

From a medical perspective, your child needs to understand the potential risks of becoming sexually active: emotional involvement, sexually transmitted diseases, and pregnancy risks. From an educational perspective, your child needs to know that sex is a wonderful part of our lives, one that should be protected and respected.

But we know firsthand that talking about sex may be much easier for some parents than it is for others. In 2010, when Jena had her third baby, her then-six-year-old son asked her how she got pregnant. Here's how she remembers her reaction:

My heart began to race. Here I was, a doctor, someone who should probably have all the right answers, but I transformed into a deer in headlights in a matter of seconds and muttered something about giving love to another person. When my son found out he had a new sister, he asked if I could hug Daddy one more time, so he could have a brother. It was then and there that I realized I had failed—not a crash-and-burn, epic fail that I couldn't recover from, but an educational fail that I needed to remedy as quickly as possible.

It was a few weeks later when I brought up the topic again. My son and I had a matter-of-fact conversation about body parts and what they do. He was completely at ease, and a lightbulb went off for me personally: If I can feel comfortable discussing sex with my children, they will be comfortable, too, no matter what age they are. Kids pick up on parents' energy, emotions, and comfort level. Parents create the climate and the attitude while doing their job of responsibly educating their children. I am happy to report that I have since engaged in many conversations about sex with my kids—and we are all better for it.

Logan's experience with this subject was very different:

When I was pregnant with my daughter, Memphis, my son, Maverick (who was almost four at the time) asked me what you needed to make a baby. I told him that you needed an egg from a woman and sperm from a man. I said that we had these "ingredients" in our bodies. I asked if he wanted to know anything else. He said no.

He didn't ask any other questions related to "sex" until one year later. We had been watching *Life*, the documentary series about the animal world on the Discovery Channel. One night, right before he was going to bed, Maverick asked me, "Mom, what would happen if Daddy put his penis in your vulva?" (Notice that he knew the word *vulva*?)

I took a breath. I felt like I was in the Sex Educators' Olympics. I asked him how or if he had ever heard of anything like that before. He said he had just thought it up in his head (probably from watching the mating scenes in the documentary). I asked him if he remembered what ingredients "made" a baby. He replied, "Sperm and egg." So I asked, "Do you know how babies typically are made?" He said no. "A man puts his penis into a woman's vulva and vagina, and that's how the sperm meets the egg. So your question was awesome. You were right. You figured it out!" He looked at me, beaming, because I had praised his question. "Do you want to know what that's called?" I asked. He replied, "Nope. That's it."

Now, we know that we are the professionals here. We don't expect that all of you have spoken to your children at such young ages, if at all. But we are telling you this in an effort to alleviate some of your anxieties. We have spoken with many parents who worry that discussing sex with their kids will encourage their children to have sex. Let us make this very clear: It just isn't true. Studies have found that not only are teenagers who have an open and honest relationship with their parents, one that includes talking about sex, more likely to delay sexual intercourse, but when they do finally engage in intercourse, they use protection. The research is on your side—talking about sex has huge health benefits for your children.

1 What is sex?

Sounds like a simple question with a simple answer, right? It should be, or at least that's what we've been telling ourselves, but it's not. When people use the word *sex*, they're typically referring to vaginal intercourse, rather than biological sex or gender—as in "We had sex the other night" or "When did you have sex?" In other words, they're talking about penis-in-vagina sex—or PIV sex, as Logan describes it to her students.

So, sure, the act of putting a penis inside a vagina is sex, but it's not the only type of sex. And it's not just for straight people. See where we're going with this? Gay and lesbian couples have sex, too. It may not be the same as your sex—or maybe it is. (We don't make assumptions about anyone's behavior.) But what we proudly proclaim is that heterosexual relationships do not own the word *sex*, even though that is what we as a culture have been implying for all these years. Sex is about more than body parts; it's about emotional and physical intimacy—regardless of people's sexual orientation—and it's as much an emotional rite of passage as it is a physical one.

If your child were to ask us what sex was, we might say that the word *sex* refers to a number of behaviors that people may engage in. Sex can be vaginal, as in when a man puts his penis into a woman's vagina; oral, as in when someone's mouth is in contact with another person's penis and testicles or vulva and vagina; or anal, as in when a penis enters a partner's anus or butt. These can be very intimate acts and come with big responsibilities, as well as the potential for pleasure.

A word to the wise: Kids ask many questions about what "counts" as sex. It is their way of evaluating what behaviors are appropriate for them and their peers. For example, lots of young people ask if masturbation is sex. Before you answer this, consider the following: Does masturbation have the potential for pleasure? Pregnancy? Sexually transmitted infections? Emotional intimacy? Think about the outcomes in order to determine your answer. While masturbation and mutual masturbation are sexual behaviors, we don't think that they qualify as sex. But feel free to disagree with us.

In the end, we want you and your children to know that there are many definitions of sex. One size definitely does not fit all. But even if your definition is all-inclusive, your children (and their friends) may not agree. So encourage your kids to challenge language and terms, too. Teach them the importance of asking for definitions before making any assumptions—because you know what they say about assuming, right?

2 **My son asked me at what age I first had sex and how I knew it was the right time. I need some advice, once someone pours a bucket of ice water over my head to revive me!**

We presume that this is not the question that you were prepared (or wanted) to answer—at least not yet. But consider it a compliment. Kids ask you because they want to use your experiences as a means of managing their own lives. Or they are curious. Or they just want to push your buttons. And, as we mentioned earlier, what kind of sex are they talking about, anyway?

This is a great opportunity for you to validate your son's question and find out why he is asking you at this particular time. You could start by saying, "Honey, that's a great question, but before I answer, I have to ask: What's up? What made you ask this?" It's important to know your child's rationale. Is he asking out of curiosity? Is he having a competition with his friends? Is he in the process of making his own decision about sex and wants your experience in order to support his choice? And, of course, before you reply with any answer, don't be afraid to turn the question back to your son: "What are *your* thoughts on this? Or when do *you* think the right time is?" Hearing the answer may help you gain a better understanding of where he is coming from, and may help you craft a better reply. As for knowing when you knew it was the right time, *did* you know? Did it turn out to be the wrong time? Is there ever really a right time? There are no absolutes when it comes to sex.

Children often think that their parents seem infallible (especially when it comes to the big issues), and that's because we present that image to them. We are often judgmental and make assumptions about our children's lives and those of their peers. But we're human, and the choices we may have made in the past are far from perfect.

Let's pretend that our decision to have sex for the first time was a brilliant one. Put that into context for your children. What was your world like? Were you in a relationship? Were you concerned about pregnancy or STIs? Had you ever had sexuality education?

Had you talked to your partner about outcomes? Ideally, all of these circumstances enabled you to make an informed decision, in which case your children could really benefit from hearing about the issues that helped to shape your choice.

But we know what you're mainly wondering: Do we think you should tell your children "when"? Our answer is, it depends. Some kids are capable of hearing personal information from you and not using it to their advantage later in adolescence. Others are not. You need to know your offspring.

We have to put on our doctor hats here for a minute, too. Any discussion about the timing of sex should also make mention of the emotional and physical elements that are intimately involved with becoming sexually active. Issues like pregnancy, sexually transmitted diseases, and emotional feelings are all important parts of the discussion (though definitely not the only ones).

As an educator, Logan is afraid that we focus too heavily on the potential negative outcomes of sex. For her, asking a group of teens to brainstorm the many outcomes of sexual experiences is extremely frustrating. While they are quick to rattle off the health "consequences," they never mention "pleasure" until she prompts them. Kids and teens must be taught that sex should be a wonderful and pleasurable experience, but all too often we focus on the dangers, rather than the benefits.

Lots of parents offer scary facts in order to curb teen sex— comments along the lines of, "If you have sex, you can die." Severe, yes. True, no. So it is far better to say, "Sex should be a wonderful part of your life at some point; however, I think its potentially negative outcomes are too hard for you to manage at this age." Sex does have many outcomes, including emotional, physical, and medical ones, yet, in an effort to protect our children, we often omit the positive ones. Our children should know about them, though, because when they do, they won't waste these experiences on unworthy partners. If you want your children to *really* listen to you, you have to be honest and balanced when you discuss sex with them.

3 My daughter's friend takes birth control pills for her acne, and now my daughter wants to know if she can take them, too.

There are many reasons why girls use birth control pills, and acne management is definitely one of them. There are others, too (we'll get to them later). As always, your daughter may be asking this question without sharing her true motive with you—not because she wants to hide something from you, but because she is not sure how you are going to react. So let's try to decipher what she may be trying to tell you:

a. *I want to go on birth control pills because I don't like my acne.*

Let's first take a look at acne and at why so many girls break out during puberty. Acne is part of puberty for both girls and boys, because of all the hormones circulating in the bloodstream. But for some girls (and women, for that matter), acne breakouts occur as hormone levels fluctuate during the menstrual cycle. It's common to experience a flare-up of acne during the week leading up to menstruation, but some people experience acne during or after their period, too.

As we've mentioned before, hormones play a role in triggering the production of sebum, or oil. Birth control pills work by lowering the amount of androgens (the hormones responsible for sebum production) in the body. Women and girls who are prescribed birth control for acne are encouraged to use other treatments (such as salicylic acid and benzoyl peroxide) as well, because the pills target only one cause of acne: oil production.

Birth control pills (oral contraceptives) may improve the complexion of some girls and women, but they're usually not the first line of treatment. They're often considered only if other treatment modalities (including other types of prescription medication) are unsuccessful. Most doctors consider birth control an option for healthy women who also need contraception.

It's important to keep in mind that not every birth control pill is approved for the treatment of acne; only certain brands are FDA sanctioned for this particular purpose, and these are all combination pills, containing a combination of estrogen and progesterone. As with any other medication, birth control has side effects, which may include breast tenderness, headaches, breakthrough bleeding, and an increased risk of blood clots. Anyone considering using birth control for acne or other reasons should talk over the decision with a medical professional and, ideally, a parent.

b. *I want to go on birth control pills because I am sexually active and need a reason other than sex to get a prescription for them.*

Take a breath. There is a chance that this is what your child is trying to tell you. We're not going to sugarcoat that. However, the fact that your daughter is coming to you looking for a way to manage her fertility is quite extraordinary. Now, as a parent you are entitled to ask her, "Are you sexually active?" In fact, you should. It's the perfect entree into a conversation about birth, sexual activity, prevention, and her partner. Sexual activity and contraception are big decisions, and as her parent, you want to make sure that your daughter is comfortable with and prepared for the way in which her relationship is progressing.

Keep in mind that birth control is not a preventative panacea for every potentially negative outcome of sex. She's still going to need to use condoms. And, as we mentioned before, there are side effects to every medication, so it's very important to have a discussion about it with your daughter and her doctor.

4 How can I explain what a blow job is to my child?

Truth be told, we still have a hard time understanding why people call the act of putting someone's mouth on someone's penis a blow job. It doesn't have anything to do with blowing, and it isn't very healthy to think of anything sexual (especially consensually sexual) as a "job." And if *we're* blabbering on about why a blow job is called that, your kids are going to be wondering the same thing, too.

So just be honest with your child. *Blow job* is a slang term for oral sex—contact between someone's mouth and a man's penis. That doesn't mean oral sex is just for men, though, as much as public discourse about it often seems to overlook the fact that women receive (and like) it, too.

Now, is that important for your child to know? Yes, but don't worry—it's not part of an insidious campaign for sexual equality. Wait, actually it is. And here's why: Even if your child has only heard the term *blow job*, chances are good that they are already aware that it has something to do with boys. If our children think that sexual pleasure and benefits are limited to males, it is impossible for them to develop healthy sexual self-esteem and maintain balance in sexual or romantic relationships. Pleasure is not just for males; as the old holiday adage says, sometimes it is better to give than to receive—or, as the new adage should go, reciprocation is always good.

The term for oral sex performed on a woman is *cunnilingus* or *going down*. Studies show that kids are engaging in oral sex probably more than their parents realize. According to a 2012 study, more than half of all teenagers ages fifteen to nineteen have engaged in oral sex, including roughly 25 percent of teens who have never had intercourse. Although very few scientific studies examine oral-sex practices specifically among middle-schoolers, there are many indications that they are on the rise among middle school and high school students. One survey revealed that roughly 30 percent (one in three) tweens (eleven to fourteen year olds) said that oral sex was part of a tween relationship. The same survey showed that among the tween group interviewed, more than 30 percent said that they know same-age peers and friends who have engaged in oral sex on more than one occasion. (Of course, there's always a chance that when teens say that they "know people" who have done something sexual, they may all be talking about the same person.) It is important to recognize that analyzing teen sex behavior has never been easy, and in the end, does it matter what everyone else is doing? We need to prep our teens to make their own independent, smart decisions.

As a medical doctor, Jena finds that the easiest part of this conversation is the one about health risks, but she still cautions parents not to sound like a textbook droning on and on about every detail of each sexually transmitted disease. If you do that, you'll notice that your child's eyes will slowly roll back in their head, and if you look closely enough, when their eyes return to center, they'll have a zombie stare and will oblige you with only an occasional nod here and there. Not good. You need to engage your child and listen, not lecture incessantly.

A common misperception among adolescents is that oral sex is not as risky as other types of sex for the transmission of sexually transmitted infections (STIs). Recent research has highlighted the fact that HPV can be transmitted through oral sex, which may lead to oral cancer. (In 2013, Michael Douglas acknowledged publicly that his throat cancer may have been caused by the transmission of HPV during oral sex.) Other diseases—such as herpes, gonorrhea, and chlamydia, among many others—can be transmitted orally as well. By making your children aware of these risks, you are arming them with information and knowledge that will hopefully empower them.

⑤ Some of my friends are getting the HPV shot for their kids. Should my child get one, too? Will they take it as a free pass to have sex?

Don't panic. This is a complex—and important—question with a complex answer that touches upon both solid science and individual parental values. But before we give you our take, we're going to give you the full rundown on HPV. If you have not yet heard about the human papillomavirus (HPV) vaccine, you likely will from your child's pediatrician. And if the doctor doesn't bring it up, you may want to. No doubt your child will hear about it from friends who may or may not get the vaccine, which was originally intended for girls and young women but is now being recommended for boys and young men by both the Centers for Disease Control and Prevention (CDC) and the American Academy of Pediatrics (AAP).

But first, what is HPV? HPV is the most common viral sexually transmitted disease in the United States. It is estimated that at least

50 percent of men and women (that's one in two!) who are sexually active are infected with HPV, according to CDC statistics. The numbers are probably even higher, however, because many people don't even realize they have HPV and/or fail to report it.

HPV is not just one virus; it is a group of viruses that includes more than one hundred different varieties. Many of these types can cause warts on different parts of the body. For example, plantar warts on the feet are caused by a specific strain of HPV, while warts that may show up on the hands and face are caused by other strains.

Among these many different strains of HPV, roughly forty types can infect the genital area, mouth, and throat and are passed along through sexual contact and/or intercourse. In many cases, the body's immune system can overcome an HPV infection before it even has the chance to create any warts, but if warts do develop, they often appear as clusters of small, flesh-colored or pink growths. Many people remark that the warts look like the small parts of a cauliflower, but sometimes they are so tiny that they are difficult to see. In women, genital warts appear most commonly on the vulva but can also show up inside the vagina, on the cervix (the opening to the uterus), or around the anus. In men, warts can appear on the tip or shaft of the penis, on the scrotum, or around the anus.

Genital warts can also develop in the mouth or throat of a person who has engaged in oral sex with someone who has HPV. In general, the warts are not painful, often resolve on their own, and may not require treatment unless they cause discomfort. If a person experiences any itching, burning, or pain or feelings of emotional distress, doctors can treat the warts with a variety of medications, cryotherapy, and, in some cases, surgical removal. Treatment will likely make the symptoms better and result in wart-free periods, but the warts often recur.

More significant, however, is that HPV can also cause cancer if left untreated. The vast majority of cervical cancer is caused by two specific strains of genital HPV. These two types usually do not cause warts, however, so all too often women and men don't even realize that they have acquired this potentially cancer-causing strain of HPV. These strains can also cause oral cancers (including mouth and throat), and cancers of the penis, vulva, vagina, and anus. The best way to detect and diagnose HPV in women is through an annual pap smear and, for women over thirty years old, an HPV test. At the time of this book's publication, there is no FDA-approved test to detect HPV in men.

Probably one of the most significant breakthroughs in medicine over the past decade is the HPV vaccine. It is designed to protect girls and boys against several of the most common types of HPV that can lead to cancer. The Advisory Committee on Immunization Practices (ACIP) recommends routine vaccination for girls and boys starting at the age of nine. The fact that the vaccines are most effective when administered to children before they become sexually active is the driving force behind this age minimum, but the recommendation extends to women and men up to age twenty-six.

Two vaccines are currently available: Cervarix and Gardasil. They differ slightly in their mechanism of action: In addition to cervical and other types of cancer, Gardasil protects against most genital warts and is recommended for both men and women. Cervarix targets certain strains of HPV responsible for cervical cancer and is not recommended for men.

Part of the controversy surrounding the availability of HPV vaccines is that some people are concerned that giving girls and boys this particular vaccine will lead them to take unnecessary sexual risks because they will think that it protects against all sexually transmitted infections.

A 2011 study in the *American Journal of Preventive Medicine* explored whether HPV vaccination led to an increase in "promiscuity." (Full disclosure: We really dislike that term. It implies judgment and a belief that we all share the same values about sex and relationships.) Researchers from the CDC followed 1,243 girls and young women, ages thirteen to twenty-four, once they had been vaccinated against the four most prevalent and virulent strands of HPV. When the researchers compared that group's sexual behavior with that of girls and women who did not have vaccinations, they found that the vaccinated group did not have a higher rate of sexual activity. Perhaps an even more important finding was that the girls and women the researchers followed still prioritized safer sex; in fact, the vaccinated group was more likely to use condoms than their unvaccinated counterparts.

Additionally, the study provided compelling information about parent-child communication: The girls who discussed the vaccination (why they were getting it, how it worked) with their mothers were more likely to prioritize safer sex.

The AAP recommends routine vaccination for hepatitis B, which is usually given as a series of three injections: the first at birth, the second at one to two months, and the third at six to eighteen months. What many people do not realize is that, like HPV, hepatitis B is a viral infection that can be spread through sexual contact and intercourse, among other routes of transmission. Chronic infection with hepatitis B can cause liver disease and liver cancer. Arguments against the hepatitis vaccination have never centered on the promotion of sexual activity, mainly because many people don't realize hepatitis B is a sexually transmitted disease. Some parents are concerned about the safety of these vaccines. The current recommendations for use come from ACIP, the CDC, the AAP, and the American Academy of Family Physicians. The recommendations for use of the vaccine are based on scientific data, including safety studies, that definitively point out that the benefits of HPV vaccination far outweigh any known risks. At the time of this book's publication, these vaccines' safety record is excellent.

Now the tough part: How to explain to your child why they are getting this vaccine? We believe that honesty is the best policy. Explain to your child what HPV is. Explain that some strains—especially the riskier ones—can be sexually transmitted through any sex behaviors—oral, anal, or vaginal. Gardasil and Cervarix do not prevent all sexually transmitted infections, nor do they prevent all cancers. It is our job as parents to make sure that our children know this. If you need some help, try expressing a version of the following:

> "*HPV* stands for *human papillomavirus.* It is a virus that both boys and girls and men and women can get. Some types of it can be spread through oral, anal, or vaginal sex, and it can cause genital warts or certain types of cancer. While I am not assuming that you're sexually active, the sooner we vaccinate you, the better protected you will be in the future. This shot doesn't protect you against everything, but it does prevent four of the most common strains of the virus. Whenever you choose to become sexually active, it will be important that you still use additional protection."

In general, we vaccinate our children before they can be exposed to any potential health threat. In the case of HPV vaccines, that means we vaccinate them before sexual activity. There are many things that we as parents cannot control. We can, however, control whether our children are at risk—at some point later in their life—for contracting this very, very common virus. Our final take: we will vaccinate our own sons and daughters as soon as they reach the minimum age requirement, age nine.

⑥ How will my child know how to use a condom?

Do you know how your children are going to know? You are going to show them. Yep, that's what we said. You, the parent/caregiver/grown-up who loves them, are going to teach your son (and your daughter) how to use a condom. But maybe you don't know how to do it. Maybe you don't remember. Maybe the amazing assortment of condoms in different shapes and textures confuses you. That's cool. There are lots of condom innovations these days. So we will teach you.

- Condoms are extraordinary health products. They may be small, but those little rubber sheaths can prevent us from getting some pretty nasty bugs, as well as protect against unintended pregnancy. First thing first: In order for a condom to work, you have to put it on and keep it on. And you have to put it on *before* you start to have *any* kind of sex.

- Condoms are wrapped in foil packages. Check the foil to view the expiration date. (Yes, condoms expire, but typically not until three to five years after they have been manufactured. That's a long time.)

- Use your fingers to tear open the wrapper. No sharp objects, please.

:• Condoms are rolled up. Place the rolled-up ring (with the tip up) at the head of the erect penis and roll it down the length of the erection.

:• After ejaculation, hold the condom in place and withdraw the penis from the vagina, mouth, or anus. (If you don't do this soon after ejaculation, the penis becomes flaccid and the condom can slip off.)

Other tips:

:• Store condoms in a cool, dry place (in lay terms, don't leave one baking in the sun on your car's dashboard or keep one in your freezer).

:• Check the package for an expiration date.

:• Never used oil-based lubrication with latex condoms; use water and silicone only.

Go buy some condoms (both male and female). Take them out, practice, play, and get to know them. Many parents haven't used them in a long time and may not remember what they feel like. But the most important thing to note is that condoms are without a doubt the only protection we have against STIs and pregnancy. And not only are they really good protection, but you (yes, you) can greatly influence your teen's condom use. According to studies, mothers who talk to their teens about condoms before they have had sexual intercourse make those teens three times more likely to use them the first time. And first-time condom use predicts future use; a teen who uses a condom the first time they have sex makes them twenty times more likely to use a condom every time. If you needed a reason to talk about condoms, there it is.

One last note about condoms: They are not as you might remember them. They are made to be thinner, more comfortable, and better lubricated than before. Recent research shows men and women rate sex with condoms as highly arousing and pleasurable. So don't let anyone try to tell your kids that condoms don't feel good as an excuse not to use one.

7 My child wants to know if sex is a good thing or a bad thing, and I'm not sure what to say.

Sex is a wonderful, amazing, awesome, fantastic thing. (Was that not strong enough?) We are sick and tired of people, pop culture, and politics suggesting that sex is bad, when it's not. What *is* bad is the way these same groups often portray sex as violent, exploitative, pornographic, unhealthy, and nonconsensual.

But keep in mind that your children have probably learned (and not through you) that sex is bad or dirty or scary. Think about it: On any given night, *The Good Wife*, *Law & Order: SVU*, and *CSI* (of any city) have provided our children with lots of material about sexual assault, rape, and abuse—not to mention the hypersexualization of young tween and teen stars in programming geared specifically toward those age groups on the Disney Channel, *The X Factor*, or *Real World/Road Rules Challenge*, to name just a few. Your kids are being hit over the head with images suggesting what they should look like and what parts of their body they should emphasize, and that they can derive self-worth from all that is outward and physical.

Of all these pop-culture portrayals, we find the images of assault, rape, and abuse the most disturbing. We don't like that the first images of sex for our young people are within the context of rape. We want young people to see loving, consensual acts of sex, not criminal ones "ripped from the headlines."

We believe that it is part of our job as parents to reframe these images and to redesign the conversation. Jena used to think that shielding her oldest daughter from certain television shows—like *Glee*, with its mature themes (including teenage pregnancy, domestic violence, and bi-curiosity, among many others)—was the right thing to do. They finally watched one show together, because Jena's daughter was interested in seeing the a cappella championship episode. Jena was prepared to fast-forward to the musical performance, when two female characters professed their love for each other and her daughter started asking questions about same-sex relationships.

Jena realized that this episode of *Glee* provided a fantastic platform to start a discussion with her daughter about myriad topics. Some of these topics were ones that Jena's daughter had heard about from friends or on other television shows but had never really wanted to ask about; other topics were new, but she was curious. They finished watching the season together, discussing themes ranging from bullying to ethnic stereotyping to boy-girl, boy-boy, and girl-girl relationships to the meaning of love and commitment. Many *Glee* subplots depicted the main characters trying to resolve moral conflicts by applying their own values. It was a great time for Jena to mention her personal values in these contexts and to explain what she would do if she faced these issues.

Jena and her daughter also spoke about sex. They spoke about mature, loving, respectful, reciprocal relationships. They spoke about self-esteem, body image, and self-worth. Jena told her daughter that her body and her health should always be at the top of her list. They discussed one of the characters, who accidentally got pregnant—the decisions she made, and what she might have done differently to protect herself against pregnancy and STIs. Jena did most of the talking, but her daughter talked, too, and when she did, Jena listened to her as best she could, with the hope that her daughter would continue talking to her for many years to come.

Logan believes it is our responsibility as parents, caregivers, educators, and doctors to present a holistic view of sex, an image that incorporates the emotional, physical, relational, and political implications and outcomes. Ideally, sex of any kind is a positive and intimate experience shared by people who care for and respect each other.

Logan's father always spoke about sex in a positive light when she was growing up; he told her and her sister that sex is supposed to be wonderful. (We know—it's not something that we assume fathers tell their daughters, though we should be changing that stereotype.) Logan's dad never told his children that they shouldn't have sex; he said that they should do it when they wanted to, not because someone was pressuring them, and that they should always be emotionally and physically protected. And those paternal messages worked for Logan—she didn't have sexual intercourse until she was eighteen years old. She knew how good it was supposed to be, and she didn't want to share it with just anyone.

Yet there's another aspect of the good/bad debate that all of us can learn from. It's called being literate—in this case, sexually literate and media literate. We need to be checking in with our kids to see how they view sex. Chances are, the images that they have seen are quite different than what we would like them to be in real life. Consider posing the following questions to your children to gauge their sexual literacy:

- How do you see sex portrayed on TV, in movies, or online?

- Do you and your friends see sex as a good thing or a bad thing?

- How does the media (mis)represent teen relationships and sex?

- Under what circumstances do fictional characters engage in sexual behaviors? (Are they drunk? Is it consensual? Are they in a relationship, or have they just met?)

Then start watching the shows your kids watch. In addition to being highly addictive, some of them grossly misrepresent the way teens act in the real world. And don't even get us started on *Jersey Shore* or *Buckwild*. Thankfully, both of these shows have now been canceled, but replacements will surely crop up.

8 My son wants to know if there is such a thing as butt sex or ear sex.

Thanks to the television show *Family Guy*, an entire generation of young people believes that if you add the word *sex* after a body part's name, it is possible for penetration to occur there. Like ear sex or belly button sex or foot sex. Ridiculous? Yes. Take it up with Seth MacFarlane. Logan, for one, is exhausted from explaining to her students that *Family Guy* isn't a good substitute for sex education.

Contrary to our personal requests, *Family Guy* isn't going away anytime soon, so we are left to answer semi-asinine questions like "Can you put your penis in someone's ear?"

Ask your kids to brainstorm what other terms have *sex* in them. They will probably come up with *oral sex*, *anal sex*, *phone sex*, and *cyber-sex*, just to rattle off a few. While some of those can be penetrative sexual behaviors, not all of them are. Phone and cyber-sex include descriptions of sexual content but don't necessarily lead to physical activity with a partner.

As with anything else, ask your children where this question comes from. Was it motivated by a television show? Was it something that they've heard from friends? In pornography? The impetus for asking the question is as important as the answer itself, because it gives you insight into what your kids have been exposed to or what their friends have been talking about.

9 My daughter asked me if she needs to be in love to have sex, and I said yes. What would you say?

We get it. As parents, we want our children to have sex under the best possible circumstances. We want them to know how to evaluate their relationships (even their friendships), and we want to give them clear examples of what that means. (Have no fear—we will talk about that later.) But you don't want to have the one child who thinks that sex magically happens when there is love. Not all loving relationships lead to sex; sex can happen in non-"loving" and not Facebook-official relationships, too.

Bear with us for a moment. This is where your personal values come into play. It's not about us; it's about you. You might tell your children some variation of, "You don't have to be in love, but I believe that you should be," or you may want to say, "Sex is best when it involves complete trust and mutual respect." It's really up to you to guide the direction in which you want this conversation to go. But it's complicated, because, as we mentioned earlier, sex can encompass a range of behaviors. Do you have to be in love to do any (or all) of those things? Think about that right now, even if your child hasn't brought up the issue of sex or love. Get your values and belief systems (and those of your parenting partner, if you have one) in check. Be prepared for when your child does initiate this conversation or when you feel it's necessary to do so. The better armed we are with our own values, the easier it is to translate them for our children.

⑩ My daughter has heard about Plan B and has many questions about how it works. How can I explain it to her?

You may hear Plan B called by another name: the morning-after pill. But, in addition to being a misnomer, that sounds sort of judgmental. So, for our purposes, we are going to call it what it is: emergency contraception (EC). EC is designed to prevent pregnancy after unprotected sex. These pills contain high doses of the same hormones found in birth control pills. They work by interacting with the hormones in a female's reproductive system to prevent the ovaries from releasing an egg. If no egg is present, fertilization cannot take place. In addition to preventing ovulation, emergency contraception may prevent fertilization and attachment to the uterine wall. While EC may aid in pregnancy prevention, it does not offer any protection against sexually transmitted infections or HIV.

In order for EC to be most effective, it should be taken as soon as possible after unprotected sex; women do not need to wait until the "morning after." Studies show that emergency contraception is most effective if taken within seventy-two hours of a sexual encounter, but newer research has shown that it can prevent a pregnancy when used up to five days after sex. If you are already pregnant, emergency contraception will not work.

EC is sometimes confused with RU-486, which is commonly referred to as the "abortion pill," but these two pills are completely different. Plan B helps prevent a pregnancy, while RU-486 interferes with the hormones necessary to maintain a pregnancy.

You probably know that Plan B has spent considerable time in the news. As of August 1, 2013, emergency contraception is available over the counter (without a prescription) for anyone who needs it. This topic was heavily debated in the media, but let us alleviate any concerns you may have. Plan B is a medication like any other. If we teach our children to respect pharmaceuticals and not abuse them or use them incorrectly, there is no reason to worry about the accessibility of EC.

We should explain to our children that emergency contraception is supposed to be used *in case of emergency*. It should not be used as primary contraception. When we hear that someone has taken Plan B multiple times with the same partner, we consider that a major relationship red flag. It's not about the pill; it's about the couple.

PART 2:

RELATIONSHIPS 101

N AVIGATING RELATIONSHIPS IS difficult, no matter how young or old you are. As adults, we may find it easy to minimize our children's experiences by chalking them up to "young love" or things that they'll "get over." There's a reason for this tactic—parents want to protect their kids and soften the blows that come from an unrequited crush—but we don't support it. Relationships (which can be friendships, romantic or sexual partnerships, or any isolated interaction between two people) seem even more challenging these days. Consider what it would be like to be fifteen again, experiencing new feelings of love (or lust), the pressure to fit in with your peers, the accessibility of social media, the inability to determine what should be public and private, and the age-old (and quite tired) sexual double standard. Would you ever want to go through that again? We wouldn't. However, given that all of these challenges are at work, our responsibility to help our children evaluate their relationships (platonic or otherwise) is even greater.

1 **My daughter was talking to a group of her classmates the other day, and some of them called her a slut. Why would they say that?**

If there were ever a word that we wish would disappear from our vocabulary entirely, it's *slut*. It is perhaps the most vicious term to describe girls and women, a term that is unmatched when it comes to degrading one's sexuality. Ask your children if there are words that are meant to negate or shame male sexuality. (*Man whore* doesn't count; adding *man* to a word doesn't validate it.) They will probably come up with *player* or *pimp*, but those words do not have the same connotation. They never will. This is what we know as (drum roll, please) the sexual double standard. This is the system that says when it comes to sex and sexuality, boys and girls (and, by extension, men and women) are not entitled to the same freedoms. It is the system that we, as both moms and professionals, seek to deconstruct (and ideally destroy).

Our society uses the word slut in a number of contexts. The following are two of those uses, as well as our counterpoint to them:

:• A girl who hooks up a lot. The brilliance of the phrase *hooking up* is that it is completely ambiguous. It can mean any type of sex, it can mean kissing (with or without tongue), it can mean meeting up and hanging out. Judging someone for hooking up is ridiculous, because

we have absolutely no idea what that person has (or
has not) done. Most (if not all) of what we know about
our friends' experiences is based on gossip. In fact, no
one shares every detail of their sexual or romantic life,
because it is intimate and personal. More importantly,
who cares? What is right for one person may not be
right for another, but who are we to judge that? As
moms (forget our doctor status for now), we want our
children to be able to hold their heads high and own
whatever decision they make about dating or any physical behavior—whether they decide to engage or to say
no. We want our children to avoid judging others and
to spend more time holding themselves accountable for
their actions. It is easy to name-call others when you are
insecure about yourself. But that's what we do, right?
We label people to make ourselves feel better. That is
not a lesson we are willing to pass down to our children.

:• A girl who dresses provocatively. Let us be clear: What
you wear does not have anything to do with what you
may do (or not do) with your body. Wearing a short
skirt or a low-cut shirt does not mean (and has never
meant) that you have indiscriminate sex. Think about
those archaic and misogynistic responses to rape allega-
tions: What was she wearing? (As if a woman asks for it
if she dresses provocatively.) If that response makes you

sick, as it does us, then it is never okay to call someone a slut because of what she wears. In a world where girls are told in less-than-subtle ways that they have to look a certain way, it amazes us that girls can still be comfortable in their own skin. Now, do we have a culture that sexualizes children and makes them want to be "sexy"? Yes. But we cannot link behavior to clothing. It does far more harm than good.

Sometimes we hear girls calling each other sluts in hopes that the term will seem endearing. "Oh, you're such a slut [*giggle*]." No. That's not endearing—it's passive-aggressive at best. We beg you to challenge your children's language so they can avoid this kind of pitfall.

❷ My child just asked me, "When did you start to date?" What is he really trying to say?

Your son might as well be telling you, *There's someone I like, and I want to go out with her, okay?* A kid typically doesn't ask this unless they are starting to become interested in a peer or if their sex-ed teacher told her class to go home and initiate conversations about "growing up" with a loved one—something Logan often encourages her own classes to do.

There are many reasons why this "homework" is important. While making parents cringe seems like a fun preteen activity, it does have benefits. If your child can start a conversation about dating with you, it is a sign of maturity. Also, while we understand that parents and caregivers alike are stressed about and swamped with a million other tasks, it is your responsibility to talk about these issues with your kids. Every parent drops the ball sometimes, but it's a giant wake-up call when your child looks at you and says (not necessarily in these words), "Listen, there are things that we need to talk about."

We need to talk about dating (or, as Christopher Lloyd told Michael J. Fox at the end of *Back to the Future*, "It's your kids, Marty. We've got to talk about your kids!"). Like everything else in the last few decades, the concept of dating has changed. It seems like the days of picking someone up and meeting a date's parent(s) are over, and that's sad, because dating protocol should be steeped in respect. It should be executed with maturity and politeness. You should need to pick someone up at their front door. Think that sounds old-fashioned? Maybe it does, but we have no problem with that label as it relates to dating. We also have no problem with young people dating in general, but we find it challenging for a relationship to evolve in a respectful way when it doesn't start with respect. If a child is taking someone to the movies or out for a hot chocolate, we want them to show up at their date's door and say hello to the parents. Don't you want that when it's your own child being picked up? Don't you want someone to respect the dating process (and your child) enough to meet you?

LOGAN'S GUIDELINES FOR DATING READINESS

You can ask someone out or tell them that you like them face-to-face. You cannot text it. I will bend the rules slightly for iChat or Skype if you don't get a chance to see someone in person regularly, but if you go to school with someone, face-to-face is the only way.

You are prepared to deal with rejection. (I remember spending an entire weekend crying to The Jets' "Make It Real" because a boy named Matthew told me that he didn't like me as a girlfriend.) Rejection sucks. It will never not suck. But handling that disappointment is a sign of maturity.

You don't measure social success by having a boyfriend or girlfriend. You don't play with someone's feelings in order to gain social status. Some people are ready for dating; others are not. It is not a race. Everyone catches up in the end.

BUT, OF COURSE, that assumes that our children will be "dating" in the way in which we once defined it. However, those days seem to have come and gone. Dating today often appears to be more of a group activity where people meet en masse and partner up. In a way, it seems like the natural extension of a Facebook-based adolescent world. Recently, a girlfriend of Jena's dropped her thirteen-year-old son off at a movie theater to meet up with a girl on what he described as "not a date." He texted on his phone the entire car ride, and when she dropped him off, his mom noticed about five other girls and three of her son's friends congregating outside the theater. She stayed in the parking lot—out of sight, of course—to make sure they all entered the theater.

Everything is for the group; nothing is really for the individual. We do things to be seen by others, not intimately. In fact, it almost seems emotionally safer for young people in date en masse because they don't have to handle rejection if they are hanging out in a group. But that's feigned emotional safety. Feelings are feelings, and crushes (as we mentioned earlier) can be completely overwhelming. Besides, Facebook shouldn't be the model for dating—ever.

③ My daughter just asked me how she'll know when she's in a good relationship. What should I tell her?

Kids need to learn how to trust their gut, as do parents, when it comes to identifying healthy relationship. So before we tackle the health of our adolescents' relationships, why don't we take a good look at our own first? It is nearly impossible for us to teach our young people about healthy relationships if we aren't exactly great role models in that department.

Sorry, but that's the truth. We can't expect our kids to abide by our relationship advice if we don't follow our own. You think your kids don't see those little things we try to hide from them? Whether we like it or not, they see all. Listen, we are far from perfect and will not pretend that we always fight fairly or that we don't fly off the handle at the smallest transgression. We have been known to lose our cool on occasion (maybe even more than that), but we are acutely aware that our children are watching or listening, and we are prepared to apologize or forgive accordingly.

But imagine how hard it is for a teen to know if they are in a good relationship; they are often too overwhelmed by being in *any* relationship. As adolescence is characterized by both a need for independence and a need to fit in, how can they determine the quality of their relationship or know whether they would even do anything about it if they found out their relationship was less than satisfying?

In good relationships, we don't worry about all the little things. We trust our partners, we feel good about ourselves, we don't worry if our partners are texting other girls or boys with certain intentions. Sure, that's easy for us to say. But our point is, if you don't feel a sense of happiness in your relationship, if you don't find your voice is being heard or that your boundaries are being respected, if being with someone makes you feel more insecure than being without a partner, well, the relationship is definitely not a good one. More importantly, it is one that you should be getting out of. We don't need to tell our kids that their relationship is bad (not unless you want them to tune you out), but we can give them the criteria for evaluating the quality of the one that they are in.

Good relationships are healthy relationships, but we're not just talking about physical health here—we mean emotional health, too. The qualities that make up a good relationship may vary from person to person, but there are some universal criteria that you can easily discuss with your child. A relationship should always make both parties feel safe, cared for, and good about themselves. Feel free to tailor your list. You can even create a list with your child; it's a great place to begin this conversation.

For us, healthy relationships should be filled with:

- Trust. This is a quintessential feature of all relationships, no matter how old or young you are. Having faith that your partner has your best interests in mind and trusting that your feelings for each other match up are important components of a good relationship.

- Reciprocity and equality on all levels. One party should not dominate the relationship or call all the shots. Things should be balanced fairly in all aspects of the relationship.

- Respect for each other's feelings, bodies, and boundaries are crucial in a good and healthy relationship. Hearing and listening to each other, and treating each other the way you would treat your best friend, are all parts of respecting each other as individuals.

- Honesty. Telling the truth, admitting when you are wrong, and being open to another person's ideas and feelings is another important component of a healthy relationship.

∴ Good communication is a key ingredient in a healthy relationship and one we all struggle with periodically. Being able to speak openly about your feelings, without the fear of being judged, and being able to amicably resolve disagreements are examples of good communication skills.

JENA'S GUIDELINES FOR SAFE AND HEALTHY DATING

The characteristics of your dating relationship should be similar to other healthy relationships in your life and should be based on mutual respect, trust, and good communication.

Spending all of your time with your partner, even if you feel like you want to, isn't always the best idea. Maintaining your own identity and interests and other relationships allows both of you to foster your individuality, which is part of healthy growth and development.

You should *never* feel pressured to do anything you don't feel comfortable with. On the flip side, you should never pressure anyone else. Open and honest communication is a key ingredient in a safe and healthy relationship.

Sometimes being in a group is okay, especially if you're just getting to know someone. I recommend telling at least one friend and your parents whom you are going out with and where you are going. Taking your cell phone on a date is important, too, in case you need to reach someone.

4 **My son's girlfriend wants him to call her all the time.**
She keeps checking up on him. Is that normal?

No, needing to monitor someone's location is not a normal part of a healthy relationship. Given *Maury*, *Cheaters*, and the dozens of other reality-based shows that "catch" people up to no good, it's not surprising that we all feel jealous sometimes. In some ways, we are told that we should always be suspicious of the people in our life. However, we must not subscribe to that school of thought.

One of the classes Logan teaches is about evaluating healthy relationships. She poses the following question to her students: "If you could create the perfect relationship, what qualities would it have?" She finds it distressing that in 90 percent of those workshops, the students' first response is "Someone who doesn't cheat." How freaking sad is that? Our young people are growing up in a world that teaches them to expect cheating. Think we're making a leap here? Think again. Our tabloid culture perpetuates the notion that celebrities jump in and out of bed with each other all the time. It seems as if no one is faithful to their partner. Can you even name more than five Hollywood couples who have managed to stay together for the long haul?

And in many cases, the consequence for cheating is nil, except for more publicity and fame. Even the cheated-on party often looks like they bounce back with little problem. As we know, though, real life doesn't work that way. We get the relationships that we demand, and if we don't speak up about our needs, we will never get what we want—and our children will never get what *they* want.

Still, jealousy is a part of life. If you think back to your own teen relationships (whatever that word means to you), remember how powerful those feelings were if you experienced them. They are all-consuming and can quickly turn someone into an insecure, emotional, suspicious mess. Young love should not be like that.

So your son should ask himself: What is the difference between basic curiosity and the need to check up on one's partner at every given moment? Control. And it's far from healthy; it's abusive.

It's also an insidious change. When someone you love (or are infatuated with, as teens often are) calls or texts you all day long, you think it's sweet. *She loves me. He needs me. He can't be without me. Oh, it's really love.* Sounds corny, yes. But think like a teen. This type of behavior can sometimes be confused for strong feelings of caring and attachment. We've spoken to some kids who even think it's flattering.

Then something happens. What seemed like undying love turns to control. It's an annoyance. It feels invasive. Excessive jealousy and controlling behavior are not signs of affection. This type of behavior is unhealthy and can be dangerous. Keep in mind that "destructive" relationships don't have to be violent, and often aren't. This scenario can be tricky for parents, because their son or daughter may not recognize the behavior as dangerous and may just feel intensely cared for by their boyfriend or girlfriend. Signs of destructive behaviors include always checking in, blaming everything on the other person, a lack of good communication skills, and a resistance to taking responsibility for one's behavior. Sometimes the controlling person tries to distance the other person from their support system, friends, and family members who have their best interests in mind.

This can be a challenging issue for any parent. Relationships are hard to decipher even when they are healthy. The idea of being controlled by a boyfriend or girlfriend may be difficult for a child to recognize and fully understand. When approaching your child about this type of relationship, we recommend discussing the basics of any healthy relationship first: mutual respect, honesty, trust, caring, and so on.

According to Teens Experiencing Abusive Relationships (TEAR), an organization set up to highlight different types of abuse in tween and teen relationships, the difference between healthy and abusive relationships is that in healthy relationships, the couple works toward the relationship equally. Healthy relationships consist of a system of checks and balances combined with equality, individuality, and compromise. In an abusive relationship, one partner takes advantage of these goals and uses them against their partner as a way to manipulate them into doing what they want. Usually there is little compromise and forced inequality, and your individuality is taken from you.

If you feel that your child is in a controlling relationship, explain to them that a line should be drawn when their freedom gets limited. Discuss healthy and unhealthy relationships. Ask them to give you examples (even if they are from pop culture) of relationships that appear "healthy" and those that do not. This is a great litmus test for you: You can see how your child perceives relationship health and where you may need to help them further. Studies indicate that less than 25 percent of teens have discussed abusive relationships and dating violence with their parents. We encourage you to help increase that percentage.

5 Should my child give a girlfriend or boyfriend the password to their email and/or Facebook account?

No, no, no, no, and no. Are we clear?

Seriously, there is no reason for a partner (for a friend, even) to have the password to someone else's email or Facebook, Twitter, or any other social-media account. No one other than a parent/ caregiver should be checking up on a teen.

But let's think like an emotional, hormonal, madly in love (or lust) teen: *I love my boyfriend/girlfriend. I want him/her to trust me. We share everything. What's the big deal?* In your child's mind, sharing passwords is as intimate as sharing your body. If you loved someone enough to be physical (and that may or may not include sex), why wouldn't you share your password? Sounds innocuous enough. But, unfortunately, it's a huge deal. If someone has access to your social media or email pages, they have control of you. They can control your posts, your communication, and the way in which you represent yourself. No one should have the ability to control who you are or how the world perceives you.

In a 2011 study, the Pew Research Center's Internet & American Life Project revealed that one in three online teens reported sharing one of their passwords with a girlfriend or boyfriend. There were some significant gender and age differences, too. Online girls were much more likely than online boys to share passwords with friends or significant others, and older kids (ages fourteen to seventeen) were more likely to share than younger ones.

In a 2012 *New York Times* article entitled "Young, in Love and Sharing Everything, Including a Password," the author discusses the negative effects of sharing passwords, including the potential for obsessive monitoring of a girlfriend's or boyfriend's account for cheating signs, and the ability to damage the other person's reputation after a breakup.

In this digital age in which privacy is almost obsolete, we think part of our job as parents is helping our kids create meaningful boundaries. Facebook and email passwords should be part of those parameters. These self-imposed limits will help your child maintain a sense of independence and individuality. Email messages and Facebook posts are meant for your child only, not for a girlfriend or boyfriend. Not only is this sense of privacy essential from a basic rights perspective, but it is healthy for all parties involved. When there is trust and respect in a relationship, partners don't need to manage each other's lives.

6 My daughter and her boyfriend don't talk; they just text. Is that weird?

Just between us grown-ups, we wouldn't say it's weird—we would say it's frightening that your daughter could call someone a (romantic) boyfriend or girlfriend but not talk face-to-face. Isn't that what "going out" means in elementary school? Logan had a "boyfriend" in the fifth grade. His name was Howard and the only time they spoke was when he (and his friend) called her (and her friend) to ask if she wanted to "go out" with him. And that was it. Dating. No more talking after that. Until they had to break up and call each other (on the phone) and say, "I don't think we should go out anymore."

In fifth grade, that makes sense. For the most part, dating doesn't really mean anything, or at least it didn't when we were children. And that was a different era. We can't tell you how many adults we have spoken to who are concerned for this generation—concerned that interpersonal skills aren't being developed properly, concerned that our kids are growing up too dependent on gadgets, concerned that tweens and teenagers can't look a person in the eye when they speak. It's as if everyone's head is stuck looking down all the time. We're not convinced that this generation of kids will be able to hold their own in a conversation or handle unprompted social interactions unless we encourage them to interact face-to-face.

A few summers ago, Jena had to speak to her daughter's high school-age summer-camp counselor because she was concerned

that the counselor and her fellow staff weren't appropriately supervising the kids; they were too busy supervising their phones.
During the entire conversation, the young woman didn't make any
eye contact with Jena. She didn't know how to handle conflict face-
to-face and opted instead to avoid looking a parent in the eye.

If you (and this applies to all of us, regardless of age) are in a
relationship with someone (and at this point, we will use the term
relationship very loosely), *you cannot just text*. If you cannot talk
to someone you're dating, then you shouldn't be dating that person
in the first place. That's the rule. Vulnerability is part of being in
a relationship, so if you can't put your feelings out there in person, then you aren't ready to be in a relationship. And not being
"ready" isn't a negative. We will all be ready at some point, and it
will make the experience that much better.

7 My son wants to know why his girlfriend calls him names when they fight.

Because she's a crappy girlfriend. Was that too harsh? That's our
gut reaction, but that may not be helpful, so let's try a different
tactic. Teen relationships are passionate, fleeting, desperate, overwhelming, tumultuous—qualities that are entertaining if you are
watching this couple on the big (or small) screen but torturous to
observe if any of the characters live in your own home.

We just called this girlfriend crappy—but that's between us. There is no doubt that a teen will stay in a relationship just to spite you if they feel like you don't understand (even if they know you are right). How do we know this? Logan did it. When she was in high school, she knew that her relationship was moving from loving and respectful to emotionally unstable and unhealthy, but the more her parents pushed her to end it, the more she tried to make things work. She told herself that her parents didn't understand what young love was, but in actuality they did—they've been together since high school.

When we get involved in a judgmental way, our kids shut us out. We need to play the game by their rules. And let us just say that even though we may have been asked what to do about name calling, it doesn't mean that our kids really want to know what we think. It's tricky, this parenting thing.

Bitch. Slut. Douchebag. Whore. We don't care what age you are—no one should be calling you names. No one who cares about and respects you should ever make you feel badly about yourself.

We need to teach our children how to fight fairly, and name calling is not fair. It is nasty, and disrespectful and speaks volumes about who you are as a person. Fighting fairly means talking about how you are feeling, saying how and why someone hurt you or offended you, and never making anyone feel ashamed of who they are or what they have done in life.

Remember how we said that respect is an important part of any healthy relationship? Name calling shows an inherent lack of respect and can be a slippery slope into verbal abuse. If your child is in a relationship with someone who consistently name-calls, it is important to engage them in a constructive conversation to address the issue. Any negative words meant to shame, criticize, mock, or put down are unacceptable.

Sometimes this type of behavior can be more insidious or harder to identify. Some people couch their damaging words in constructive criticism, but if it becomes habitual, the effect can be the same. It not only is unhealthy but can have long-term effects on a person's self-esteem and emotional well-being. It can also set the stage for relationships in the future. If your child is in this type of relationship as a young person, he/she may feel this is the norm and seek out other, similar relationships in the future.

8 My daughter confessed that her friend has an abusive partner. She doesn't know how to help her friend, and she wants my advice.

We are big on honesty, and we want you to know that you don't need to feel pressured about parenting "the right way." There is no such thing. While that has always been our philosophy, there are some alarming trends when it comes to dating-related violence and abusive relationships. We share this not to frighten you (as you have hopefully picked up by now that we are not alarmists) but so you will realize that you hold the power to change the statistics.

Your input can dramatically affect the health of your child's relationships. So please, before you panic, keep that in mind as you read the following information.

According to a 2000 study conducted by Teenage Research Unlimited and sponsored by Liz Claiborne Inc.:

- One in three teenagers reports knowing a friend or peer who has been hit, punched, kicked, slapped, choked, or physically hurt by their partner.

- One in four teenage girls who have been in relationships reveals that she has been pressured to perform oral sex or engage in intercourse.

- More than one in four teenage girls in a relationship (26 percent) reports enduring repeated verbal abuse.

- 73 percent of teens said they would turn to a friend for help if they were trapped in an abusive relationship, but only 33 percent who have been in or known about an abusive relationship said they have told anyone about it.

- Nearly 80 percent of girls who have been physically abused in their intimate relationships continue to date their abuser.

The following are some warning signs that a person is in an abusive relationship, according to the National Teen Dating Violence Prevention Initiative. This person:

:• has undergone a dramatic change in weight, appearance, and/or grades since they started seeing this person.

:• worries about how this partner will react to things they say or do.

:• feels that their needs and desires come second to the other person's.

:• thinks twice about expressing their own thoughts and feelings.

:• worries that they might make the "wrong" decision about what to wear, where to go, and whom to hang out with.

:• has family members or friends who warn them about this partner or worry about their safety.

:• is frightened of this partner—maybe not before, but lately.

Okay, you're probably freaking out. You're right; this is awful news. But if you teach your children to value themselves over their relationship status, if you make them feel smart and beautiful and worthy of love and respect, then they will be less likely to find themselves in this kind of unhealthy relationship.

9 **I hear my kids using the word "rape" in a joking, humorous way that makes me uncomfortable. How should I best put an end to that?**

There is nothing funny about rape and our kids need to be made aware of that, immediately. Rape isn't sex; it is a crime. That's a tough thing for teens to understand. To be sex, the experience must (we repeat, must) be consensual.

Consent is a word that applies not only to sex, but everything else in our lives. Our children should recognize that it is important to ask permission (and get it), before they do anything; and of course, equally as crucial is respecting someone's "no," if indeed they get that response, too.

Here are some guidelines that all of us should follow:

:• Consent is non-negotiable.

:• You always have the right to say yes; you always have the right to say no.

:• Not saying no isn't the same as a yes.

:• Never assume anything, even if someone has given you permission before.

It is important for us to remember that rape and assault aren't just women's issues. Many boys and men don't report their assaults or rapes because we have some archaic (and plain asinine) idea that someone is less of a man if they are raped. Not only is this line of thinking incorrect, but incredibly damaging to all parties, of all genders and orientations.

PART 3:

SEXUAL ORIENTATION

W E REALLY WANTED to introduce this chapter to you with "Not all of us are heterosexual. No big surprise. Let's move on," but we had a feeling that might not be sufficient for you. So let's try something else. Sexual orientation is a person's innate attraction (physical or emotional) to another person. Young people today are far better equipped to (and far more progressive in how they) accept the many sexual orientations that exist. But that doesn't stop us, as parents, from being confused about how to broach these issues with our children or how to combat some of the intolerance and homophobia that still exist today.

❶ My child asked me if I think he's gay. How should I respond?

We are thrilled that a child would feel comfortable asking this question of his parent(s). Think about what it was like when you grew up—could you have asked this? How would your parents have responded? There is something very refreshing about a child being able to talk about an issue that many families would once have seen as shameful or embarrassing.

Regardless, you cannot answer this question—at least, not in the way in which your child is asking you to, because we cannot label other's sexual orientations. Here's why: Sexual orientation refers to the people we find ourselves attracted to—our own gender (gay or lesbian), the other gender (straight or heterosexual), or both genders (bisexual). Attraction is that feeling deep inside that draws us to another person. It is not a choice; it is not a conscious decision. It is just who we are.

Logan uses the following analogy to explain this dynamic:

Think about your first crush. How did you know that you liked that person? Did you wake up one day and decide you would begin that day to have feelings for that particular person, or did your body and heart decide for you? Your head doesn't make the choice; your heart does. This is the same reason why we talked about inconvenient crushes in chapter 1. We don't always like the person who makes sense. Parents, think about your past relationships. No, *really* think about them. Did you always date the safe choice? Of course not. Now, we are by no means comparing being gay to being unsafe. What we are saying is that falling in love or lust is not a decision you make with your brain.

Now that we've said that, behavior and identity are two completely different issues. Brace yourself—this is where it gets confusing. In Indiana University's 2010 National Survey of Sexual Health and Behaviors (NSSHB), which was the largest sex and behavior study of the last few decades, 7 percent of women and 8 percent of men identified as gay, lesbian, or bisexual. However, 15 percent of people said that they had had sexual experiences with someone of their own gender.

See what we mean? Behaviors do not dictate your identity. Sexual orientation is about your feelings, not about what you do with your body. But what does all of this really mean for you? Your child is asking a few questions here. He is probably saying, *How do I know if I am gay? Are you still going to love me if I am gay? Is there something wrong with me?*

The first thing you should be asking your child is, "Do *you* think you're gay?" and, "What makes you think you may be gay?" Does he have a crush? Did someone at school call him gay? Is it because he wears pink? The answers will give you clues about why your son approached you with this question in the first place.

As for whether your son is actually gay, it can take years for people to figure out who they are. Some children know early on that they are gay or lesbian; others identify as gay much later on in their lives. Puberty is a time when we start to make sense of those feelings, but even so, many children and teens have some same-sex sexual experience. It may be masturbation; it may be kissing, touching, and so on. Same-sex experimentation doesn't automatically make someone gay. Sexual orientation isn't about what you do; it's about how you feel.

As parents, we should provide our children with unconditional love. Their sexual orientation shouldn't change that. We also need to make sure that we are on the same page with our co-parents so that our children feel loved no matter whom they are attracted to.

② How can I best explain gay marriage to my child?

When we speak about gay marriage, we are really talking about civil rights—the right for two people to formally join their lives together; the right to have a family and a relationship that the US government recognizes; the right for couples who have the same genitals to have the same freedoms as couples who don't. As we write this, thirteen states allow gay marriage and key passages of the Defense of Marriage Act have been declared unconstitutional. A cultural shift is at play; the United States is changing.

One day, while Logan and her three-year-old daughter, Memphis, were playing with princess dolls, she implied that a princess needed to marry a prince. Logan told her that princesses could marry whomever they loved, and they didn't always have to love a prince. Sometimes they could love and marry another princess (or even a commoner). "Really?" Memphis asked. "Can two girls get married?" Logan told her yes. Memphis then declared that she would marry Logan. "Mommy, then we'll get married." And Logan agreed. She decided to save the conversation about why parents can't marry their children for another day.

Kids are naturally open-minded. We color the world for them. As parents, we need to watch what we say and how we say it. Feel free to initiate a conversation with your kids about gay rights, marriage, and family when you see it on television or in movies—it's a great springboard for discussions about many other subjects.

Jena used to discourage her kids from watching some of the television programs with more "mature" themes. Now she takes every possible opportunity to discuss all of these issues as openly as possible. It's amazing how an episode of *Modern Family* can spark a lively and thoughtful dinner conversation. Seeing certain issues unfold on TV has allowed her kids to speak freely and question openly.

As parents, we need to think consciously about what gay marriage is about. It's the right for a family to exist. It's a couple's right to have their love recognized. In a world where there is so much hate, violence, and abuse, shouldn't we be prioritizing love above all else?

❸ I was driving my son's friends in a carpool the other day, and they kept using the phrase *that's so gay*. My brother is gay, and my son told me he feels uncomfortable when his friends say this, but he didn't speak up. Should I encourage him to?

We are huge proponents of not just having a voice but using it. In this case, your child should absolutely speak up.

Think about the way people use the word *gay*. When someone calls something gay, is it used as a positive term or as an insult? It's the latter—calling something gay has insidious homophobic undertones, even if that wasn't a child's intention. While the original definition of *gay* was *happy*, today it refers to a huge population of people.

We believe that it is important for children to understand that words have power. Encourage them to start a dialogue with their friends and ask them to consider what would happen if they were calling something "gay" and a friend who may actually be homosexual (or who has a gay parent or relative or friend) walked by. How would they feel? Pretty crappy, probably. Calling attention to this kind of thing can have very positive effects on everyone. Your son is standing up for what he believes in and, at the same time, giving his friends the ability to practice empathy and see things from someone else's perspective.

Using the word *gay* in an inappropriate or mean-spirited way is an insidious form of bullying. If we don't teach our children to challenge it, they wind up implicitly condoning it. We also believe that if a child's friend makes fun of him because he speaks out against using this homophobic phrase, he needs to know that this not a friend you want him to have. A good friend never makes us feel badly for doing the right thing.

❹ I caught my daughter and her friend comparing their vulvas. Does that mean she's gay?

If we had a dollar for every time we compared body parts with a friend (even as adults), we'd be able to buy at least thirty lattes. Kids often assume that looking at someone's body (even if that person is the same sex) is a sign of homosexuality. Obviously, it isn't. As your child's body is changing, she is desperate to know whether her development is "normal." Kids and teens often compare body parts in an effort to see how they measure up, or simply out of sheer curiosity.

Jena's girlfriend once walked in on her seven-year-old daughter playing "doctor" with a friend, and, very upset, she called Jena on the phone for advice. "I think they were looking at each other, and they closed the door, so they obviously knew what they were doing was wrong," she said. Before Jena could say anything, the friend continued: "I don't know what to do—it's so inappropriate."

Jena jumped in at that point: "Listen, sexual exploration is a normal and healthy part of sexual development. Your daughter, like so many other children this age, is developing a healthy relationship with her body and her sexuality. The way you handle this situation can have ramifications down the line. If you barge in on her, tell her that what she is doing is inappropriate, and make her feel guilty about exploring her sexuality in the safety and comfort of her own home, she may hide her sexual questions and exploration from you in the future. Take this opportunity to support her in becoming a happy, healthy, strong person whose sexuality will continue to develop whether you like it or not."

5 I think my son's best friend is gay but doesn't realize it. Should I say something?

What were you planning on saying? Do you want to "out" this child before he officially identifies as gay? *If* he even identifies himself as gay? Do you want this information (which may or may not be accurate) to color how your son now views this friendship?

We don't believe that this should ever be a conversation about a particular child or teen. We should be explaining to our children that they will have many friends in their lives who are different from them, whether those differences are based on race, religion, sexual orientation, or gender.

Parents are the strongest role models for their children's friendships, especially during the school-age years. We recommend discussing with and showing your child the important aspects of friendship: loyalty, commitment, devotion, and respect. It's so important to give them a sense of independence in choosing and maintaining friendships and to celebrate diversity among their peers.

⑥ My daughter wants to know why some people do not like gay people. Any suggestions?

We have always found that the toughest questions to answer are the ones about why people hurt or hate others. For us, talking about sex is easy, but talking about homophobia or racism or gender biases or religious persecution is very difficult. How do we explain ignorance and intolerance in a way that makes sense, when it doesn't even make sense to us?

Our children need to understand that most hatred in this world comes from ignorance. It is sometimes easier for a person to hate instead of taking the time to learn about someone or something that is different. Though, of course, this idea does not excuse the behaviors. Unfortunately, homophobia and prejudice against lesbians and gay men are widespread in the United States. And, despite some progress, discrimination and hatred remain.

As with many aspects of parenting, teaching your child to understand this can be very challenging. Studies tell us that children respond best when they have a strong, secure foundation from which to act, and that starts with us. Open and honest communication, encouragement, and positive role models are the best ways to ensure that children are comfortable enough in their life to stand up for themselves and for others.

At one get-together that Jena attended with her kids, a friend's husband made an off-color remark about gay men playing football. A few people laughed, and while the comment definitely went over Jena's son's head, her daughter seemed uncomfortable about it. As hard as it was to say something in a large crowd and in front of this man's family, Jena knew she had to speak up. She informed her friend's husband that anyone can be a good athlete, no matter what their sexual orientation is, and she knew she had done the right thing for her children and for others.

It's not always easy to explain hatred and discrimination to children, but we need to be careful about what we say, how we act, and what types of jokes we make or let slide in front of them. They are listening to us, and they are learning from us what is appropriate and what isn't. Homophobia, racism, and hatred of different cultural or ethnic groups usually stem from the same place of ignorance, intolerance, and fear of being different. These are not the qualities that any of us should want to foster in our children. You are doing them a great service if you teach and show them from an early age to honor and respect their own differences and those of the people around them.

PART 4:

GENDER AND GENDER IDENTITY

G ENDER—THE STATE OF being female or male—is something
many of us don't give a second thought to. Most of us wake
up and feel secure that our sense of self and gender is in sync with
our body (or, more specifically, our biological sex). That's not true
for everyone, however. Gender is complicated, and gender identity
even more so, for some people.

Perhaps what makes this subject even more complex is that our
expectations of what it means to be male or female are often based
on old ideas of what is "masculine" or "feminine," and these ideas
change from culture to culture. The fact is, there is no one way to
experience and express gender.

**1 My son just told me that he doesn't feel like a typical
boy. Does that mean he's gay?**

What does it mean to be a "typical" boy? Is it all about sports
and toughness and the color blue? Sure, sometimes it seems that
way. But there is no such thing as typical when it comes to gender.
Stereotypical, yes, but that's about it.

The media throw around different terms related to this subject,
often mixing them up or completely misrepresenting them. So let's
break them down:

:• **Sex** refers to a person's biological sex and includes their sexual and reproductive organs, hormones, and genes.

:• **Gender** is part of a broader, sociocultural context and refers to how society thinks we should act as girls and boys, women and men.

:• **Gender identity** is defined by our personal feelings about and/or inner sense of our own gender. Studies show that gender identity usually develops during early childhood and can be shaped by parents, society, and a number of other biological factors.

:• **Sexual orientation** describes emotional, romantic, and/or sexual attraction for people of the opposite gender, the same gender, or both genders. "Acting like" a boy or a girl has nothing to do with sexual orientation. Expressing masculinity and/or femininity has to do with your own gender, not whom you are attracted to. In addition, the way we express gender is based on stereotypes anyway, so we struggle (both as mothers and as doctors) with this idea that there is anything "typical" about boyhood or girlhood.

While we're on this topic, let's revisit Toenail-gate. Toenail-gate, as Jon Stewart coined it on *The Daily Show*, was a raging media discussion about a J.Crew catalog photo in 2011. Sound familiar? In the image, Jenna Lyons, J.Crew's president and creative director, is painting her five-year-old son's toes neon pink. It is a beautiful picture of a mother and son, both of them giggling candidly. The caption under the photo reads: *Lucky for me, I ended up with a boy whose favorite color is pink. Toenail painting is way more fun in neon.*

Logan loved this photo for two reasons: It was a refreshing look at a parent and child, and at that very moment, her own six-year-old son's toenails were painted neon pink. But the innocent image incited rage among conservative-news outlets. Fox News's psychiatrist, Dr. Keith Ablow, told Lyons (in a public message) to save money for therapy because her son would need it after this toenail-painting scandal. He also said that showing a boy with pink toenails was part of an insidious campaign to support the transgender agenda. And (take a breath—if you're anything like us, you're feeling your own rage now) Ablow even posited that boys who wear pink early on will question their gender identity later in life. WTF!

We couldn't help but wonder: If the ad had featured a little girl wearing navy blue and a football helmet, would it have garnered the same negative attention? We think not.

Don't want to take our word for it? Think back to a time when you didn't wear societally mandated pink or blue as a child. Are you now questioning whether you are male or female? This is one of the dumbest statements of all time. Colors do not have genders. Toys do not have genders. Nor do they cause us to question our own.

Let's have a brief history lesson, shall we? Until right before World War I, there was no "rule" about colors and gender. In fact, the majority of clothes for boys and girls were white dresses. It was a matter of practicality. White could be bleached. Dresses made diaper changing easier. Then the infant-clothing industry and related stores stepped into the conversation and proposed that pink (yes, pink) was a more suitable color for boys. Blue was "daintier" and thus better suited to girls. By the 1970s, the feminist movement helped to bring gender-neutral clothes back. However, this was clearly short-lived. According to Jo B. Paoletti, author of *Pink and Blue: Telling the Girls from the Boys in America* (2012), gender-specific clothing as we know it today came about in the 1980s, with prenatal testing and great consumerism. Her point is, our reliance on the pink–blue binary isn't based on anything sexual at all. It's about marketing, plain and simple.

Our children's gender will develop naturally as part of who they are and has nothing to do with whether a mother puts pink, blue, or polka-dot nail polish on them. And playful explorations have little to do with determining a person's sexual orientation.

The concept of being a "typical" anything is bullshit. It limits our ability to express ourselves by confining us to a particular box or color. Now ask yourself when you last allowed your son or daughter to wear something that wasn't "typical." Sure, girls have greater freedom in this area, but the point is that there has never been one way to be a boy or a girl.

Research does reveal that there are gender preferences in the way some kids like to play. Both of us can attest to this pattern in our own children, but neither of us feels comfortable attributing all of these differences to a penis or a vulva. The fact is, there is a wide range of kids who don't fit neatly into any category, and that is simply not a cause for concern.

2 **All of my daughter's friends are into boys, but she isn't yet. She recently asked me if she's a lesbian, and I'm not sure what to say.**

Remember that time when you could almost feel the hormones in the air, that time when everyone around you was buzzing, when spring fever happened every day? If you were in the throes of those sensations, they consumed your life. We remember the crushes, the note passing (or, today, the text messaging), the waiting in hallways to see if you "accidentally" bumped into the person you liked. If you were one of the many people *not* going through this experience, you thought your overly hormonal peers were acting like idiots or you felt left out. Sometimes you felt a little of both.

Jena remembers this time vividly. As the youngest child with two older brothers, she always had a large group of male friends. When her girlfriends started developing crushes (and vice versa), she didn't look at the boys the same way. They were still her friends—nothing more, nothing less. When Jena's best friend, who happened to be a boy, asked her to go to the movies alone, Jena was confused. She didn't have those feelings for him, and he was left as perplexed as she was. Jena's romantic feelings toward boys didn't develop until almost two years later; she was slightly behind the curve, compared with her peers. She still rejects the old *When Harry Met Sally* rule that men and women can't be friends.

This time can be confusing if you are figuring out (or have already figured out) that you are gay or lesbian, or if you're not interested in broadcasting your feelings out loud via social networking. As parents, we need to support the individual needs of our children, but in the case of this particular question, we also need to have more information.

To help your daughter make sense of her feelings, you can always say, "It may seem like everyone is into boys, but I can assure you that not everyone is. Not everyone is having crushes right now, and not all of those crushes are on people of the other gender. When you are ready to 'like' someone, it will happen. But only you know if you are a lesbian. I don't know who you are attracted to; the only person who knows that is you. Are you attracted to girls?"

This can be a complicated time for boys and girls. Many are trying to figure out who they are and are using their peers as a measuring stick. And their classmates may be developing at different paces. Raging hormones, societal and peer pressure, and a fear of being different can cause many kids to question themselves physically, emotionally, and sexually. It can be challenging to feel left behind or different than everyone else. The most important thing we can do as parents is to support our children and to let them know that we accept them unconditionally. This encouragement will give them the strength to figure things out over time.

3 My son told me that he doesn't feel comfortable in his own skin and that he feels that he should have been born a girl—that he really *is* a girl. Help! I'm at a total loss.

Let's see if we can help you to better understand what your child is saying.

According to several studies, most children develop their gender identity by the age of three. But some people's gender identity doesn't match up with their physical body. Their outside body may be physically male or female, but inside they really feel like the other sex. The following terms may apply:

:• *Transgender* refers to people whose gender identification doesn't match with their biological sex.

:• *Cisgender* or *cis* refers to people whose perception of their gender matches their biological sex.

:• *Gender nonconforming* refers to people who do not follow traditional or expected sociological expressions of gender. While all transgender people are gender nonconforming, not all people who are gender nonconforming are transgender.

No matter what label applies, your children are going to be true to themselves regardless of biological sex. Some children know very early that their personal gender identity doesn't match up with their assigned gender. Other children struggle with it for decades. For parents, this can be incredibly challenging. No one expects their son or daughter to feel uncomfortable with their biological sex or to be transgender. But for some families, this is a reality.

If you're reading this in search of answers about your own child, wondering if your child is indeed transgender, we may not be able to advise you. The answer may not be apparent right away, but the picture may become clearer and clearer as your child gets older. We've spoken with some parents who have told us that their child consistently expressed dissatisfaction with their assigned gender, while other parents couldn't identify any set pattern in this regard.

Identity conflicts need to continue over a period of time to be classified as a gender identity disorder (GID), a formal diagnosis by mental-health professionals. We find this term a bit misleading, because we do not view identity conflicts as disordered behavior, but the clinical diagnosis defines GID as a condition in which a male or female feels a strong identification with the opposite sex. A person with GID may feel a conflict between their physical sex and the gender they identify with. According to statistics from the US National Library of Medicine, most people recognize that they have an issue with gender identity before they reach adolescence, and this "disorder" occurs more often in males than in females.

The symptoms of GID can vary by age and by person. Some people may cross-dress, while others may want sex-change surgery. Some people privately identify more with the other gender but do not verbalize these thoughts and desires.

In children, some of the more common symptoms may include:

:• A belief that they will grow up and become the other sex

:• Consistent verbalization of a desire to be the other sex

:• Feelings of disgust toward their genitals

:• Feelings of rejection by same-sex peers

:• Depression/anxiety

In older teens and adults, some of the more common symptoms may include:

:• A desire to live as a person of the other sex or gender

:• Feelings of isolation, depression, or anxiety

:• Presenting or dressing as a different gender

:• Withdrawal from social interaction and activity

:• A desire to get rid of their genitals

In order for someone to receive a GID diagnosis, that person's feelings of being the "wrong" (again, not our choice of word) gender have to persist for at least two years. The diagnosis is most often made by a psychologist or a psychiatrist after a thorough medical and physical exam. GID is not the same as homosexuality; a person with GID may be attracted to partners of the same and/ or opposite sex.

We highly recommend individual and family counseling for children who are grappling with gender-identity issues. Oftentimes, kids suffer from feelings of isolation, stress, anxiety, and depression can help address these issues and improve self-esteem through therapy. As parents, we ultimately want our children to feel good about themselves and comfortable in their own skin, so having a mental-health professional work alongside your family can encourage positive affirmation and reinforcement.

4 My child just asked me why some people have surgery to become another sex. How should I explain this to him?

As we mentioned, not everyone identifies with their biological sex. For some transgender people, problems of poor self-esteem, depression, and anxiety may arise, especially at the onset of puberty or other gendered biological milestones. Of course, some of this anxiety and wavering self-esteem may be due to cultural factors, too. There are a wide variety of support measures available for people struggling with these issues, some of whom opt for hormone and surgical treatment to suppress their biological sex characteristics and gain the characteristics of the opposite sex.

The surgery is called gender reassignment surgery and involves a series of surgical procedures and hormonal medical treatments. Because it is irreversible, people who choose to have this surgery go through an elaborate screening process to make sure they are 100 percent certain that this is what they want.

We always believe that children (of all ages) deserve honest answers to their questions. And while discussing the *T* in *LGBT* may be difficult for some, the fact is, it is a great conversation to have with the young people in your life. There is much more to gender than what is between our legs.

⑤ There's a show on television called *RuPaul's Drag Race* where men dress up and compete as women. Are those men transgender?

We love that RuPaul has made her way back into pop culture. When we were teens, RuPaul had a pop hit called "Supermodel," and now, almost twenty years later, she has a televised drag show. This is a great question, even though it may feel like a complicated one. If you've explained the concept of transgenderism to your children, it is not surprising that they may be confused by *Drag Race* (or any other show with drag characters). But in this case, men who dress up in women's clothing for the purposes of entertainment are not transgender—they are called drag queens. They don't identify as women; they identify as men. Sometimes we call people who get pleasure from dressing in the clothes of another gender transvestites or cross-dressers.

But cross-dressing brings up an interesting issue: We as a society are fairly limiting about how we express gender, especially for cisgender boys. We don't give individuals a great deal of freedom. Consider how few pink clothes there are for boys (of all ages) and the range of styles and articles of clothing available in the girls' sections of stores.

Jena had a friend whose husband once flipped out when he caught his four-year-old son putting on his mother's makeup and walking around the room in her high heels. He was so worried about what his son was doing, he ended up yelling at him and sending him to his room. Jena's girlfriend got upset at her husband for making such a big deal about what she viewed as harmless activities. As kids explore, learn, and grow, yelling at them only hurts their sense of self and their self-esteem. This husband revealed his own biases and insecurities instead of recognizing his son's expressiveness and curiosity.

PART 5:
SEX, SEXUALITY, AND PREGNANCY

P REGNANCY CAN BE either one of the most wonderful or one of the most horrifying experiences a woman has. (Don't get mad at us for the "horrifying" remark—Logan threw up every day for nineteen weeks during both of her pregnancies.) Pregnancy is one of those topics that both fascinates and confuses many of us. It seems as if the myths about pregnancy that we heard as teenagers still permeate teen conversations today. We are committed to dispelling these myths and initiating some new discussions about contraception, family planning, and reproductive technology.

1 After health class, I overheard my daughter talking to her friends about a video they watched. They were wondering aloud if you can get pregnant the first time you have sex. Should I bring this up?

Yes, absolutely. You can acknowledge that you heard (but weren't eavesdropping on—this is a very important point!) the conversation your daughter had with her friends. You can explain to her that myths about first-time sex have been around since you were young. In fact, most sex myths have spanned many generations.

We've heard from many boys and girls who have watched outdated puberty videos in health class, accompanied by little follow-up discussion. Many are left with unanswered questions, so this is a great time for you to jump in with the facts. A girl can become pregnant the first time she has sex. Anytime a girl has vaginal intercourse with a boy, she can get pregnant. It's important for boys and girls to realize that even if a boy or man ejaculates outside the vaginal canal or "pulls out" before he ejaculates, a girl or woman can get pregnant. When we were in high school, our peers used to call withdrawal the "pull and pray" method, because there were no guarantees.

Information about withdrawal today is still confusing. Like all other birth control methods, pulling out is more effective if it's done correctly—that is, before ejaculation. Experienced couples who have more self-control may be able to utilize this method more effectively, but even if the guy pulls out in time, a pregnancy may happen. Some research shows that pre-ejaculate (or pre-cum) can pick up enough sperm left in the urethra from a previous ejaculation to cause a pregnancy. According to statistics from Planned Parenthood, of every one hundred women whose partners use withdrawal, four will become pregnant each year if they always do it correctly. Of every one hundred women whose partners use withdrawal, twenty-seven will become pregnant each year if they don't always do it correctly. Withdrawal also does not protect against sexually transmitted diseases. For people having sex, condoms must be used to protect against the transmission of infection.

You'd be surprised how much misinformation is out there and
what your child may or may not know. We strongly believe in
sex education, but, unfortunately, not every school offers a comprehensive, up-to-date program—and that's where we recommend
you come in, by initiating a basic, matter-of-fact discussion with
your child about how pregnancy occurs. Here's a review:

Anytime a girl and a boy have sexual intercourse, pregnancy
is a possibility; the only requirements are one sperm and an egg.
It doesn't matter if intercourse takes place in a bed, in a pool,
standing up, or lying down. Location and position are not relevant
either; once a girl begins to menstruate, pregnancy is possible. It's
important to note that some adolescent girls who have never had
their period could still potentially ovulate (release an egg) and
then, if they have sex, get pregnant. This scenario is very rare but
not impossible.

After the start of menstruation every month, a girl's pituitary
gland secretes hormones that trigger the ovaries to release an egg.
For many people, ovulation occurs in the middle of the menstrual
cycle (at day fourteen, if the person has a twenty-eight-day cycle).
However, keep in mind that menstruation is prone to quite a bit of
variation: some women have longer cycles, some women ovulate
earlier or later than the middle of their cycle, and ovulation can
vary among cycles in an individual.

After the egg is released, it takes a trip into the fallopian tube,
where it waits patiently (about twenty-four hours) for fertilization
from a single sperm. Studies have shown that sperm can survive for

up to three to five days, so there is a sizable window for fertilization. If the egg gets fertilized, it moves into the uterus and attaches itself to the uterine lining, where it begins to grow into a fetus.

② My son asked me if a girl can get pregnant from oral sex. What should I tell him?

While you may be shocked that your child posed this question to you, try not to worry. It's a good question, and many of our own students have wondered the same thing.

The answer is simple: No, it's not possible to get pregnant from oral sex. In order for a girl or woman to get pregnant, sperm must enter the vagina and make its way through the cervix, and the fallopian tubes and eventually into the uterus. But while you're discussing this with your son, it's worth mentioning that although pregnancy isn't possible, getting a sexually transmitted infection is. And this last part is important. Many teens use oral sex as a means of experimenting with sex and sexual feelings without engaging in what they see as "sex." As we mentioned earlier, sex shouldn't be limited to intercourse, no matter what past presidents have said.

Regardless of definitions, it would be remiss of us to ignore the concept of protected oral sex. Yes, *protected* oral sex. We know that may seem counterintuitive—our students have implied (or flat-out announced) as much—but oral sex can come with risks that, if it's practiced in a smart way, can be managed and reduced with condoms and dental dams. Latex condoms (which come both in flavors and unlubricated) can be used as protection during what the kids call "blow jobs" (we're kidding, obviously). Dental dams—polyurethane or latex sheets that can be placed on a woman's vulva so that her partner's mouth doesn't make direct contact with the genitals—can be used to prevent the spread of STIs when oral sex is performed on a female. The fact that dental dams are not widely available makes this an interesting discussion about gender, sexuality, and equality, too.

③ Are there people who can't get pregnant?

Think of the people you surround yourself with. Chances are, not all of them have children. Some may have chosen not to parent, while others may have been diagnosed with different types of infertility, some of which were preventable. There are many reasons why couples are infertile—the quality and quantity of a man's sperm, hormonal issues, endometriosis, scarring of the reproductive system caused by an untreated sexually transmitted infection, among many other causes—or infertility may be situational.

4 **My child asked me how gay couples have babies. What should I say?**

Actually, there's a lot to say. Logan often asks students to determine the recipe for making a baby. There are two ingredients and one baking source: sperm, egg, and uterus. How those three join together depends on the couple. So, needless to say, the options available to gay and lesbian parents are broader today than ever before. Here's a quick look at some of the most popular approaches:

:• **Adoption:** This can include joint adoption by a same-sex couple, adoption by one partner of the other's biological child, or single-parent adoption. In the United States, certain states allow for full-joint adoption by same-sex couples.

:• **Donor insemination:** A man donates his sperm—most commonly through a sperm bank or fertility clinic—in order to fertilize an egg.

:• **Co-parenting:** A parenting situation where the parents aren't married. This is sometimes an option for couples who may not be in a romantic relationship (e.g., a lesbian and a gay man) but want to team up to have children. They often share custody and responsibility for the child.

But co-parenting is certainly not limited to gay or lesbian couples; heterosexual couples do this, too.

:• **Surrogacy**: A woman has a baby for a couple who can't have a child themselves. Some gay men opt to donate sperm to a surrogate, in order to establish a biological relationship with the child. Sometimes a surrogate uses her own egg, but many times a donor egg is used.

⑤ My kids read a magazine article about a pregnant man and now have a lot of questions. How can I explain whether pregnancy is possible in men?

This question is a little more complicated than you might think. The short answer is no—biologically speaking, women carry babies. The female body is genetically engineered for this miraculous task, so seeing images of a man carrying a child can be very confusing to your own kids. But if you've covered issues of gender with your child, this is easier to tackle. Thomas Beatie, "the pregnant man," was born biologically female, but his gender identity was male. Though he lived his life as a man, he still had a uterus, and that enabled him to get pregnant.

If you have a budding scientist on your hands, you may want to offer additional information. We know through science that a human fetus can develop to term in an environment other than a uterus. For example, ectopic pregnancies or abdominal pregnancies are possible, but they aren't safe and can be life-threatening. However, at some point in the future, reproductive biologists may figure out how to how to maintain a pregnancy outside the uterus (which currently sounds more like a sci-fi movie than a reality) and thereby give men a chance to carry a child, too.

6 **I have twins, a son and a daughter. I know that I'm supposed to take my daughter to the gynecologist at some point, but what about my son? Should I take him to see anyone special?**

We've been asked this question many times, because most parents are understandably confused. Let's start with the girls. The American Congress of Obstetricians and Gynecologists (ACOG) recommends that the first gynecological visit take place sometime between the ages of thirteen and fifteen, or when girls become sexually active, whichever comes first. Because most girls feel nervous before their appointment, we think it is really important to find a doctor or nurse-practitioner who has experience with young women and who will take the time to make your daughter feel comfortable. This may or may not be your own gynecologist. Involve your daughter in the decision: Ask her if she prefers a man or woman. Most young women we have spoken to prefer female doctors, but some don't care. Your pediatrician may be able to recommend someone appropriate. But don't belittle your daughter's feelings. She's the one who has to feel comfortable. It doesn't matter if your doctor is amazing and delivered her into the world— it's not about you; it's about her.

Giving your daughter as much information as possible will empower her and provide her with a stronger comfort level during the process. On the whole, the first visit rarely includes a pelvic exam, unless your daughter has a specific complaint. The doctor will most likely ask you to leave the room, which is both okay and important.

One of Logan's sixteen-year-old students wanted to have a private conversation with her doctor about contraception and STI testing. No matter how hard the daughter tried to accomplish this goal, her mother refused to leave the room, and thus ensured only one outcome: Her daughter never got the health care and support that she needed. Don't be that parent! Leave the room and let your child develop her own relationship with her doctor.

Your daughter's first visit to a gynecologist will most likely include a physical exam and a breast exam; as she gets older and/ or becomes sexually active, a pelvic exam, a pap smear, and STI testing will also become routine. We think it's vital for your daughter to develop a positive relationship with her health care provider. She needs someone to whom she can ask questions about her changing body, menstruation, sexuality, and healthy lifestyles, especially if she feels uncomfortable speaking about these issues with you. (Yes, that's hard to hear, but teens do need privacy. And think about it: You really don't want to know all the details of their intimate life, do you?)

Keep in mind that many girls see a gynecologist long before they become sexually active, for reasons such as yeast and urinary tract infections, or even a labial jellyfish sting. (Seriously, this happened to one of us. Delivering a baby was less painful.)

When it comes to boys, many of them continue to see a pediatrician until they leave for college; however, some prefer an internist or a family doctor. We've spoken to boys who got tired of kiddie toys and animal wallpaper and felt like they needed a more "grown-up" office; others don't care. Pediatricians are trained to address puberty and teenage issues. But, as we mentioned for the girls, it is equally important for the boys to feel comfortable with their doctor so they can address any issue in a confidential and supportive environment. Because the HPV vaccine is now recommended for boys, they should have a full physical (including a genital exam) and be tested for STIs, too, if they are sexually active.

This is the time when your children build the foundation for future interactions with medical providers. Think about what you would like from your doctors, and help your children find the person who is best for them.

7 **My son asked me if teen pregnancy is really common. What should I say to him? I'm not sure that I know the exact answer.**

We are always amazed by the mass amount of sensationalism in the media when it comes to teenagers and sex. Scary headlines and jaw-dropping statistics are often used to get the attention of parents across the country. These scare tactics work, but they are actually doing you a disservice, because not only are you worried, but you may not even be getting the right information.

When it comes to adolescent pregnancy, you might be surprised to hear that the rates have dropped to historic lows in the United States. According to data released by the Centers for Disease Control and Prevention in the most recent Annual Summary of Vital Statistics, the number of teen births across all groups has declined dramatically. According to many experts, the declines are attributable mostly to the increased use of condoms.

Teenage pregnancy certainly remains a challenging issue, though. Studies report that children ages twelve to fourteen are more likely than other age groups to have unplanned sexual intercourse and are more likely to be coerced or "talked into" having sex. Other statistics show us that up to 66 percent (two in three) adolescent pregnancies occur in teenagers who are eighteen and nineteen years old. Notable risk factors that increase a girl's chance of becoming pregnant in her teens include socioeconomic disadvantage, an older male partner, single or teen parents, ethnicity (especially non-Hispanic black, Hispanic/Latino, and Native American), and poor academic performance.

Studies consistently demonstrate that knowledge-based programs that focus on teaching kids about their bodies, about birth control, and about how to prevent sexually transmitted infections help decrease teen pregnancy rates. The best programs are those that provide medically accurate information about contraception, condoms, and abstinence and encourage critical-thinking skills.

A word to the wise, though: It is very easy to rely on the shaming of teen moms in order to get your point across. We feel strongly that this is the wrong tactic. First, it is unfair to hold young women to different standards than we do young men. Second, we do not know the circumstances under which some teen moms have gotten pregnant. Third, many teen moms out there are working exceedingly hard at providing and caring for their children. For these reasons, we must not lump all young mothers into one group.

8 **My thirteen-year-old daughter and her friends like to watch *Teen Mom* on MTV. Over dinner the other night, my daughter asked us why the girls never seem to consider having an abortion. I'm not sure how much information I should give her. What are your thoughts?**

Tell her the truth. And, yes, while it is important to share your values about abortion, you must—we repeat, *must*—also give her the value-free truth. While the jury is still out on how these shows impact our culture and teen pregnancy in general, the fact still remains that they provide you with a tremendous opportunity to engage in a dialogue with your children.

And despite the hype in the news and the abundance of shows just like *Teen Mom*, the rate of teenage pregnancy in the United States is at an all-time low. Still, there are many teenagers who have sexual intercourse, and some do opt to get an abortion, regardless of how few media representations of that there are. And in case you are worried that providing information to your daughter about safe sex, pregnancy, and abortion will in any way increase her chances of getting pregnant, let us assuage your fears: Several studies claim just the opposite.

Differing opinions about pregnancy termination are widespread. While we respect that, we're going to be completely transparent: Our belief is that the decision to continue a pregnancy or to end it is solely up to the girl or woman who is pregnant. It is her body and her decision. And regardless of our values (or those of others), abortions are very safe medical procedures.

That said, the type of abortion that occurs depends upon how far along a pregnancy is. There are two ways to induce an abortion: medical and surgical. Most abortions are performed within the first twelve weeks of pregnancy (and the earlier the decision is made, the easier the procedure is).

A medical abortion involves the use of medications that will most likely cause the body to bleed. The bleeding can last up to two weeks, and it is extremely important to follow up with a doctor to make sure the abortion is complete. Many women compare the bleeding that they experience to a very heavy period. Medical abortions can be performed up to sixty-three days after the first day of a woman's last menstrual cycle.

A surgical abortion involves the use of surgical instruments. In early abortions, the cervix is numbed and the embryo is removed through a narrow suction tube. The procedure usually lasts roughly ten to fifteen minutes and can be performed in a clinic, doctor's office, or hospital, usually under local anesthesia. Surgical abortions should be performed only by a qualified physician.

The type of abortion a woman has depends on several factors, including how long she has been pregnant and her personal preference. If a girl is under the age of eighteen, her parents may or may not need to give consent, depending on what state she lives in. Planned Parenthood provides a list of states and their requirements at www .plannedparenthood.org/health-topics/parental-consent-notification-laws-25268.htm.

It would be remiss of us not to acknowledge how very personal (and very political) the issue of abortion is. Wherever you live, you have a responsibility to know the laws in your respective state, because those laws matter—to you, to your daughters, and to your sons and their potential partners. Options are important, despite the sad fact that some states have greatly reduced them.

3

Emotional and Mental Health

DOES YOUR TEENAGER often seem tired, depressed, with-drawn, or anything other than fine? Does he alternately yell at you and ignore you? Are you ready for a refund for your one-way ticket on the teenage emotional roller coaster from hell?

There is no doubt that emotions are heightened during puberty. Your teen is trying to maintain some independence from you but still wants to be part of a group of their peers. Add to that the pressure of crushes, dating, and rejection, and you have a pretty wound-up kid. Maybe your child is just going through that phase of puberty where no one understands and everything is quite dramatic—or maybe they really are depressed. How can a parent tell?

In this chapter, we'll tackle some of these big issues. One of parents' biggest challenges during this time is deciphering the normal and not-normal parts of puberty. For example, depression in children can look different than it does in adults, and sometimes it's not so easy to diagnose, so it's important to be aware of the warning signs.

It's also important to put yourselves in your children's shoes. Do you remember being grounded? Lying on your bed, listening to music for hours? While you may or may not consciously remember that time, your child's moodiness may trigger your own emotions, resulting in a less-than-optimal conversation (cue the screaming and the fireworks)—or none at all.

By giving you some advice about when you should seek further attention from a health care professional and when you should perhaps, as your child tells you, "chillax," we can get you down this rocky road.

1 My son's behavior is unpredictable; he seems out of control. Help!

Let's make a list. Take a look at your son: there's hair in new places, his voice is cracking, he notices a funky smell under his arms, and he is getting erections for no apparent reason. He may be left feeling that this bus (aka puberty) is driving itself and there's little he can do to control it. He can blame all of these changes on his hormones, but as the hormones are wreaking havoc on his body, they're also doing a number on his mind.

If you think mood swings, emotions, and feeling out of control are reserved for girls, think again. The surge of emotions that comes with an increase in hormone levels during puberty is gender-neutral. And feeling out of control isn't fun for anyone. If your child is experiencing these feelings, he should find someone to talk to, engage in stress-reducing activities (like exercise or meditation), and realize that he is not alone. Everyone feels like this at one time or another.

Unfortunately, we are not in control of puberty, and that's a very difficult concept for young people to understand, just as when women are pregnant or menopausal, they're not in control either, and that's nearly impossible for them to accept even as adults. So acknowledge your child's feelings. You'll be surprised by the connection you can foster simply by validating your son's emotions. Feeling out of control can be very isolating for him; he probably feels like no one understands what he's going through. Though it can be incredibly challenging to parent through this phase, it is at this very point that your son most needs your support and understanding. Even if it seems as if having a talk with his parents is at the bottom of his list (behind doing homework), keep the lines of communication open and let him know that you are there for him if he needs to talk or vent.

This conversation may be hard to initiate, and everyone's style is slightly different. That's okay—it just needs to feel comfortable to you. The goal is to try to help your son identify his behavior and recognize its erratic nature so that together you can determine what may be triggering it.

A good rule of thumb for conversations is to always pose open-ended questions (questions that cannot be answered with a simple yes or no). Ask your son, "What do you think is going on?" or, "Why are you feeling like this?"

Sure, you're probably going to get the typical "I don't know" response. If that's his answer, now is a great time to let him know that you remember feeling this way, too. Tell him about a time when you feel like an emotional train wreck. You can assure him that he is not alone, that everyone feels the way he's feeling at one point or another. This is also a good time to encourage him to find an outlet for his emotions, such as jogging, swimming, kickboxing, meditation, or whatever he might be into at this time.

2 My daughter and I used to spend lots of time together, and she used to confide in me. Now she consistently blows me off. It seems like she doesn't want anything to do with me. Is this normal?

Your child's pursuit of independence is a normal part of development and, as hard as it is for some parents to accept, shouldn't be viewed as a rejection. Think about it: You probably did the very same thing to your parents. (Jena's mom never forgot the time Jena asked her to sit "at least ten rows" behind her and her friends at a movie theater.)

Spending less time together is not the only change that you'll notice. Your child will most likely want to spend more and more time with their friends and hibernate in their room for hours at a time, and when you are finally together as a family, your child may continue to communicate with friends through texting and so on. Your job during this phase is to remain constant and consistent. We know it doesn't feel great if your child seems embarrassed by you or speaks to you flippantly, but don't let hurt feelings get in the way; you are doing your job well if your child is trying to foster a sense of autonomy.

As you navigate these tricky times, keep in mind one of our favorite parenting quotes from Ann Landers: "It is not what you do for your children but what you have taught them to do for themselves that will make them successful human beings."

3 Why does my daughter act happy one minute and sad the next?

While we aren't fans of placing blame, we will make an exception this time: blame hormones. Though it's easy to focus on the myriad external changes that happen during puberty, just as many changes are going on inside your daughter, too. Those same hormones causing her body to grow in different directions, among other things, are sending her on what seems like a giant emotional roller coaster ride. One minute she's happy; the next she's upset, irritated, or ocscillating between different moods and emotions. And while it's not uncommon for her to feel confused or frustrated or overwhelmed about all these changes that are happening, they're completely normal.

Now, as parents, we are by no means suggesting that it is okay for our kids to scream at us or at their siblings or both. We are entitled to be treated with at least a modicum of respect, but our children should know that many of their feelings are hormone-related, and you should know that while you may want to ground your kids for an eternity, these outbursts are not entirely within their control. A lot is going on with them right now: their bodies are changing, they're feeling all these new emotions and sensations, they may be struggling with how they feel about themselves and their new bodies, they want to be accepted by their friends and not rejected by their crushes . . . The list goes on and on. Our kids need to know that we understand.

Yet while your oversensitive child may seem out of control, she can try to control her reactions. Once she recognizes that it's normal to feel this way and that everyone goes through it, you can offer her the following advice to help her ease those mood swings:

> :• **Talk to someone.** It's great to have an open and honest relationship with your parents, so talk to us; we can help you more than you probably realize. Otherwise, speak with someone else you trust: an older sibling, a friend, a coach, or a teacher. Just knowing that other

people are going through emotional upheaval or have experienced it in the past can help you deal with all of your feelings.

:• **Don't react immediately;** try to step back from a situation. If you need to, count to ten before reacting. As trite as this sounds, it really works, because it enables you to offer a more levelheaded response.

:• **Exercise.** We can't stress this enough. Even if you're not athletic, getting twenty to thirty minutes of cardiovascular exercise per day can keep your mood swings in check.

:• **Sleep.** This is very important, too. Studies have shown that sleep deprivation can exacerbate mood swings. At your age, you need about nine to ten hours of sleep per night.

:• **Release stress.** Whether you take a walk, do yoga or Pilates, talk on the phone, or watch a sitcom, you must find time each day to alleviate your stress, even if it's for only a handful of minutes. (Just be prepared for your child to throw this advice back at you when you tell her to clean her room or turn off the TV: "Mom, I need to destress!")

When Jena was fourteen, she was invited to a Bruce Springsteen concert with a few girls on her lacrosse team, who were taking the train into New York City one evening midweek. When Jena called her mom from a pay phone (remember those?) at the high school to let her in on their plans, her mother emphatically said no. (In her mom's defense, the other girls were all two years older and had tickets, while Jena was going to scalp hers.) Needless to say, Jena didn't take it well. She came home from practice and locked herself in her room, blasted Bruce Springsteen so loudly that the neighbors could hear, and threw a temper tantrum. She came out of her room only twice: the first time to let her mom know how she had ruined her social life, and the second time to use the bathroom. Both times Jena's mom ignored her, and Jena came to her senses, oh, about thirty-six hours later.

There's no real road map to this side of puberty. Teenagers face an array of emotional and social issues during this period of development that aren't really quantified in the same way as the physical changes are. So much is going on as your child is faced with questions of independence, separation, self-identity, and fostering relationships with their peers. Reactions seem to get amplified or exaggerated and often result in Academy Award–winning performances in the category of Best Actor—Puberty. The relationship between you and your child is also tested as your son or daughter strives to become self-reliant while you desperately try to maintain your relevance and some control.

Even when parents understand and accept all the factors at play, this is often a difficult period for them. Some parents have a hard time letting go of that aforementioned control; others find that part easy but worry that their child isn't old enough to make mature decisions. Most parents don't enjoy being the target of anger and defiance. As mutual frustration mounts, both parent and child can become reactive, leading to an ongoing pattern of negative interaction. We've all been there, and believe us, we feel guilty about it. We should know better; we do know better. But sometimes our children make us so damn frustrated.

Both parties need to find a better way. The key to disarming this negative spiral is to find outlets to express anger, frustration, and confusion in a productive way, rather than deny it or try to control it. The expression of anger can be healthy as long everyone is respectful. We know—easier said than done. But here are a few tips for communicating with an angry teen:

- Listen, listen, listen! As best you can, try to focus on the situation from your child's perspective.

- Don't interrupt, especially if your child is explaining their feelings. Placing blame, raising your voice, and accusing can end all communication.

- Don't belittle their feelings. Those emotions and insecurities are very real—they just can't see the big picture right now.

:• Try to stay in the present moment and stick to the facts. Bringing up past situations and emotions can make a simple conversation snowball into a throw-down. As a parent, your feelings are important, too. Express them calmly and rationally, and remember to show (and tell) your child that you care for and love them.

As hard as it is in the heat of the moment, one of our jobs as parents is to help our children gain a greater self-awareness. Angry teenagers can turn into angry adults who have a difficult time expressing themselves and their feelings. You can help your child gain control of their emotions and acquire solid communication skills by teaching them the art of self-reflection. Encourage your child to consider these questions:

:• Do I have reasonable expectations?

:• Is my anger covering up other feelings, such as fear, rejection, or sadness?

:• What types of situations make me angry? Is there a pattern?

:• Whom am I directing my anger at?

:• What are better ways to express feelings of anger?

:• Am I communicating effectively? Does my anger help me get what I want?

:• Am I controlled by my emotions, or am I in control?

It goes without saying that this dialogue is best accomplished when you and your child aren't in a conflict. Remember, it's hard not to react to someone's anger, but ultimately you want your child to be an effective communicator, even if they feel angry. Anger is universal, an emotion or a feeling; your child's behavior is a choice. One of the toughest jobs for parents is to step back from a conflict long enough to realize that you can guide your child into taking responsibility for their choices while also leading them in the direction of making good decisions.

④ My son seems really depressed. Is he just being moody? How do I know if he needs to see a doctor?

Mood swings plague all of us. You play referee between your kids for hours, you feel like you should pitch a tent in your car because you've been carpooling since dawn, you're working to meet a deadline, trying to balance everything. As we write this, we worry if we remembered to write down who is picking up our children at school on the class sign-in sheet. Your kids are dealing with their own stresses, too; add their fluctuating hormones to the mix, and you have a recipe for some serious melodrama. For parents, the challenge is to decipher between normal moodiness and clinical depression.

There's a big difference between clinical or major depression and feeling sad or down for a little while. People who are clinically depressed have persistent symptoms that can interfere with their ability to function normally, both academically and socially. If depression has become a state of mind, rather than a temporary mood, and seems to be getting in the way of your child's ability to function normally, they may have a problem.

Keep a lookout for the following symptoms, especially if your child experiences several of them for more than a few weeks:

:• Loss of interest in activities they used to like

:• Feelings of helplessness, hopelessness, or worthlessness (your child may express this verbally or make mention of these feelings in a journal, a blog, or communication with friends)

:• Constant feelings of sadness, anxiety, or "emptiness"

:• Lethargy, lack of energy, or fatigue

:• Difficulty concentrating or remembering

:• Falling grades or missed assignments

:• Changes in appetite or weight (not eating and losing weight, or eating more and gaining weight)

:• Changes in sleep patterns

:• Inability to function normally in everyday activities (sometimes manifested as lack of hygiene or failure to perform daily rituals)

:• Preoccupation with death and/or suicide

It's important to remember that everyone can be affected by depression differently. Some children have all of these symptoms; others experience just a few. The key to figuring out whether your child is clinically depressed lies in the intensity, persistence, and duration of these symptoms. If you think that your child is suffering from clinical depression, get help as soon as possible. Study after study shows that early intervention, which may include talk therapy and/or medication, can make a huge difference.

❺ My partner and I completely disapprove of one of our daughter's friends. We think she is a bad influence on our daughter. What should we do?

Considering how many kids pass in and out of your children's lives, there will more than likely be a few friends whom you don't approve of. In some cases, it may be wise to bite your tongue, because you don't want your disapproval to backfire and make this friendship more appealing. In addition, the ability to pick friends wisely and judge another person's character is a fundamental life skill that your children need to acquire. If you step in too much or too often, they may not learn these lessons for themselves.

However, sometimes it is necessary to get involved. In other cases, such as when a friend is making risky choices and exposing your child to dangerous or illegal experiences, you probably want to act. Try to voice your concerns in a nonjudgmental way, without pushing away or attacking your child. Be honest and express your feelings, but avoid labeling the friend as "bad" or "dangerous." First, this kind of comment can fuel your child's assertion of independence, giving them ammunition to deliberately choose friends that they know their parents will disapprove of. Second, your child may tell that friend that you have labeled her "bad" or "dangerous." You don't want to judge another teen, especially one who is not your own. You don't know about her living situation or what she has experienced, and when she comes to your home, you don't want to create an even more hostile environment.

Jena had a friend in middle school who shoplifted as a hobby. After the friend was caught at a local deli, Jena's parents made it clear that this wasn't a friendship that they'd like to see continuing outside of school. At first Jena objected, but after her parents expressed their concerns calmly and set firm boundaries, Jena set her own limits for the friendship. The friend eventually got help for an ongoing habit that led to some serious legal issues. Looking back, Jena realized that her parents had had her best interests at heart all along.

Logan loved going to her friend Ricki's house, where they could call boys on the phone and invite them over to hang out in Ricki's basement, because her parents never came downstairs. Adolescents' burgeoning sexuality can feel overwhelming, and they need an outlet to safely explore such new feelings. In Logan's case, Ricki's house gave her an outlet to flirt—and the potential to play Spin the Bottle. (If she can admit it, so can many of you.)

We all had friends who were probably not the best pals for us, but some, like Nicki, were more fun, whereas others, like Jena's shoplifting friend, were on the more extreme end of the spectrum of bad influences. As parents, we need to pick our battles. There is a difference between a friend who introduces your child to potentially criminal behavior and one who just opens your child's world up to new (normal) adolescent experiences. Before cutting off all ties between your child and her problematic friend, consider what else is going on. Chances are, your child knows exactly what your concerns are but is still desperate to make her own way in the world.

6 My daughter has always been a bit of a worrier, but now she seems overly anxious about school, friends, and after-school activities. How can I help her?

Anxiety and stress are common reactions to all sorts of situations your child may be facing, from midterms and report cards to performing in sports games, concerts, and school plays to getting invited to birthday parties and school dances. And while stress is not always a negative—for example, it motivates some people to meet challenges, like preparing for an exam—we need to understand how to provide our children with stress-management and relaxation techniques when they need them.

When Logan was a teenager, she would listen to music before an important test. Doing so put her in the right mind to tackle a particularly complicated task. (In case you were wondering, her tenth-grade song of choice was Annie Lennox's "Walking On Broken Glass.") Ask your children to think about what helps them to calm down. If music is their thing, they can make special playlists. For some teens, photos help. An activity that seems small or unimportant may be just the thing your children need.

If the anxiety or stress becomes so overwhelming that it gets in the way of your child's ability to function, that's known as an anxiety disorder, of which several different types exist. If your daughter is like the girl in this question, she may suffer from generalized anxiety disorder (GAD), which is characterized by constant worry or anxiety over many different activities or events. People with GAD have much more anxiety than the average person and often have a hard time making it through the day without a persistent sense of tension and worry. Kids with GAD may excel at different activities but tend to worry exceedingly about many things. This amount of anxiety usually produces some physical symptoms, including fatigue, restlessness, headaches, irritability, muscle aches, light-headedness, difficulties swallowing or breathing, and/or sleep problems.

As parents, we don't want to see our children suffer. GAD is best addressed by a health care professional who can examine your child and rule out any other potential cause for their symptoms. Once a diagnosis of GAD is established, the condition can be effectively addressed and treated. Studies have shown that people with GAD respond very well to a combination of medication and cognitive-behavioral therapy. Behavioral changes can also help.

Some people find that limiting caffeine and other potential anxiety-producing triggers, as well as learning how to cope with stress, can work wonders.

Other anxiety disorders—including panic disorder, separation anxiety, obsessive-compulsive disorder, and post-traumatic stress disorder—can be effectively managed and treated as well.

7 As soon as my son comes home from school, he goes directly to his room. Whenever I try to enter his room to talk to him, he tells me to knock first, and when I ask harmless questions about his day, he tells me that he'd like to be alone.

This pattern is pretty common. Many teenagers spend an inordinate amount of time in their rooms, coveting their privacy—sometimes away from younger siblings and other distractions (namely, you!). We need to respect our children's need for privacy, which definitely increases during adolescence, though we all need downtime at any age. (How many times during your day would you give just about anything to run to your bedroom, shut the door, and hide out indefinitely?) After a long and sometimes stressful day, your child may just need to escape to a safe place, relax away from all of the pressures of the outside world. And many teenagers who seek this kind of solace aren't really spending time "alone"; they are most likely "plugged" into cell phones, iPads, laptops and communicating with their friends via texts, emails, FaceTime, instant messaging, et cetera. It's a new world out there—being social without face-to-face (or, in reality, skin-to-skin) engagement.

While this is all normal behavior, it's no reason to disconnect entirely from your child. We recommend respecting their space. Knock first before entering their room, and tell younger siblings to do the same. Logan's dad, from the time she was a little girl on, always knocked on her door before he walked into her room, even if the door was open. It was his way of saying, *I'm here, and I respect you and your room*. It was a good mutual lesson to learn early on; he gave Logan privacy and made it clear that Logan and her sister should give their mother and him privacy, too.

But this isn't just about a room. Your child may also be asking for privacy in other areas of their life. Think about what your son is really saying when he answers the question "How was your day?" with "Fine," or what your daughter is telling you when you prompt her to describe what she did at school and she responds, "Nothing." They are letting you know that they need a little space and time to process their day before they discuss it with you.

This time to process is fairly underrated, but no child likes to be badgered with questions, especially an adolescent. When your child tells you that they want to be alone or they don't want to talk about it, just gently let them know that you're always there to listen, if they ever do want to talk. Studies show that teenagers with parents who ask questions about their day feel cared for and supported, even if they don't always want to talk right away. In our opinion, what's most important is for your children to know that the door is always open for them when they want to talk—but of course they have to knock first.

8 My child seems exhausted all the time. I'm concerned.

Your child probably *is* exhausted! It's not rare for boys and girls going through puberty to experience fatigue and exhaustion. All the physical changes and growth they're experiencing mean their bodies are in overdrive; coupled with their shifting sleep schedules and the fact that they have to get up early for school, it's no wonder they're so tired.

Children over the age of twelve should get at least nine hours of sleep, but oftentimes that isn't the case. As we mentioned in chapter 1, your child's biology and age play a large role in their sleep habits. As they progress through the teenage years, their circadian rhythms become geared to keep them awake later in the evening and to wake them up later in the morning. Unfortunately, our school districts haven't received the memo, so if your child goes to bed around ten o'clock and has to wake up at 6:30 AM or earlier, they're going to be dragging the next day.

As hard as it is to get teenagers to go to sleep (one of our favorite books of all time is *Go the F**k to Sleep*, by Adam Mansbach), we need to try to facilitate as much rest and sleep as possible. If your child's fatigue and exhaustion seem persistent despite the number of hours they are sleeping, make an appointment with a doctor to rule out the possibility of a more serious cause of fatigue, which include a chronic infection, seasonal allergies, asthma, thyroid disorders, diabetes, and anemia. A health care provider should be able to uncover the cause of fatigue in your child if it is medical in origin.

9 **Why does my daughter need to conform? I used to love her sense of independence and individuality; now she just talks, walks, and looks like her friends.**

Your child is at a vulnerable age where her need to fit in with a crowd is paramount. No one likes to feel like an outsider or get teased for being different, so the easiest thing to do is to indeed talk, walk, and look like everyone else. It would be so much better if everyone could just accept one another's differences at early ages—feelings of insecurity and the need to fit in would be much less profound. But for so many kids, unfortunately, it's not their reality, especially during early adolescence. Worse, if you don't talk to your child from an early age about respecting and prioritizing individuality, it's going to be nearly impossible for them to miraculously "get it" during adolescence.

When conformity becomes about experimentation or engaging in risky behavior that a peer group is involved with, some kids may run into trouble. Smoking, pressure to have sex, and experimentation with drugs and alcohol are some of the challenges your child may be up against. Being able to exercise good judgment and make independent choices are two skills many parents would love for their kids to harness. The question is, how can parents help their kids acquire them?

Studies show that parents who stay connected with their children throughout these years have a significant impact on their child's decision making. According to the American Academy of Pediatrics, children who are most successful at standing up to peer pressure share "three main characteristics: self-discipline (I shouldn't do this and if my parents find out, I'll be in trouble), a strong moral and ethical foundation (I shouldn't do this because it is wrong), and healthy self-esteem." Kids who lack self-esteem often have a stronger need or desire for acceptance and therefore give in to negative peer pressure more easily—with the unfortunate result that they engage in group activities that may not always be safe or healthy.

We should be giving our children examples of what individuality looks like throughout history and pop culture. Whether you like her music or not, Lady Gaga is a great example of someone who supports and encourages creativity and uniqueness. It is our responsibility to teach our children that we value them for what they can do and who they are, that their worth is not wrapped up in what they look like or whether or not they wear all black or have stepped out of the pages of a catalog. If "fitting in" is important to them, maintaining something that is just "theirs" should be equally, if not more, important. Does your child have a special activity, talent, or skill? Mastering one skill (or committing to learning one) is a fantastic way to give kids an identity outside of their school social clique, which, as we know, can be fleeting.

Jena's daughter is involved in a theater program that attracts children from all over her area. Her daughter has maintained her friendships with her fellow participants over many years. At first, driving to other towns seemed like a chore, but as time passed, Jena realized these relationships outside school were invaluable for her daughter. They gave her an outlet and provided an additional space where she could be herself among people who have known her for years, without worrying about what was "cool" or "in" or about being accepted. She was already accepted in these circles, and that took a lot of pressure off her.

10 A handful of kids are picking on my child at school. I've heard a lot about bullying on TV. Is my son being bullied? I spoke to him about it, but he doesn't want me to do anything—he's worried I will make it worse.

Unfortunately, this scenario is not uncommon. National surveys reveal that bullying is a widespread problem in many schools. According to the American Academy of Child and Adolescent Psychiatry, roughly one in two kids will experience school bullying at some point during primary or secondary school, and at least 10 percent of children are bullied on a regular basis.

One of the challenges for parents is identifying this problem. Most people have been teased or poked fun at by a sibling or friend. When it is done in a playful manner and both parties think it is funny, it is usually not harmful, but when teasing becomes spiteful, mean-spirited, and constant, it crosses the line into bullying and needs to stop.

Parents need to keep in mind that bullying can take on many forms, some more obvious than others. Bullying may involve hitting, pushing, shoving, name calling, harassment, public ridicule, and threats, but it can also involve isolation, social ostracization, and rumors. Cyber-bullying involves using social media—chat rooms, email, instant messages, Facebook, Twitter, and other social-networking sites—to hurt feelings and spread rumors. No matter what form it takes, the desired result is the same: bullying intentionally harms someone physically, emotionally, and/or socially.

Sometimes it's difficult for parents to figure out what is happening at school, especially if their child isn't communicating. Warning signs that parents should keep a lookout for include:

- A desire to change the routine (a child doesn't want to ride the bus or go to school anymore)

- Mood swings

- Change in appetite

:• Change in sleeping patterns

:• Loss of interest in activities

:• Decrease in social interactions/spending more time alone

We need to be clear with our children about what we expect from them. And this isn't just a conversation about what happens if your child is being bullied; it's also about what happens if your child *is* the bully.

One afternoon at the playground, Logan and her son, Maverick, saw a boy being chased and picked on by a group of older boys on the opposite side of the park. There were plenty of people watching, but no one did anything—except for Logan. She grabbed Maverick and ran across the field to break up the incident. "How dare you chase this child? You want to be tough? That's not tough. You never treat another person like that! I will call every one of your parents!" she yelled at them (even though she didn't know any of them or their parents).

When it was over, Logan looked at Maverick and said, "If I ever hear that you have bullied another child or treated him badly because of what he looks like or who he likes or what religion he is or anything else, I will take away every single thing you own." It was a clear message. We do not tolerate bullying—ever.

We believe that the role of the bystander is a crucial one. As they say on the New York City subways, "If you see something, say something." If your kid sees someone being bullied, they should speak up. In the worst-case scenario, if they feel scared, they should know to ask a grown-up whom they trust to intervene. If we don't teach our children to get involved, they become part of the problem.

Of course, not every childhood flare-up constitutes bullying. Most kids have been left out on the playground or picked last for an activity in gym. Logan (though she was the tallest in her class) was picked last for basketball regularly. She wasn't good at it, and her classmates knew it. In Jena's son's gym class, one of the boys got hit in the head with a dodgeball. Needless to say, he was dazed and started to cry. After the little boy composed himself, he got angry and called the boy who accidentally hit him a bully. The gym teacher had to explain that it was an accident and that what happened did not qualify as bullying.

Sure, some of these incidents can be upsetting, but they are great opportunities for our children to learn how to stand up for themselves, as well as to recognize that they may not be good at everything and that accidents can occur. These are all learning experiences.

⓫ My son told me that he hates his life and that no one would miss him if he were "gone." Should I take this seriously, or is he just trying to get my attention?

You should without a doubt take this statement 100 percent seriously. Are we clear enough? Very often, children who attempt to take their own lives have previously alluded to suicide among family and friends over and over again. A child who makes this kind of statement is crying out for help and needs a tremendous amount of love and support. If you notice self-harming behavior but your child is unwilling to talk, make sure he knows that you are there to listen when he's ready to talk. In the meantime, seek the help of a mental-health professional, especially if you think your child's behavior is the result of social issues or bullying. Let your child know you care about him; ignoring the issues is definitely not the right way to go here.

According to statistics from the National Institutes of Health, suicide was the third leading cause of death among fifteen to twenty-four year olds. Some notable gender differences presented themselves as well: Boys were five times more likely to die from suicide, but girls were more likely to make attempts. Suicide was much less common among children ages ten to fourteen, but all threats need to be taken seriously.

Children who have a history of the following may be at higher risk for suicide:

- Previous suicide attempts

- Psychological or behavioral disorders (this is especially true for boys)

- Alcohol and substance-abuse problems

- Family history of suicide

:• Gay and lesbian sexual orientation

:• Physical or sexual abuse

:• Easy access to firearms or potentially lethal medication

Being aware of the risk factors and taking all comments, threats, and suggestions seriously are important steps parents can take to help a child who is suffering from suicidal thoughts. Knowing the signs of potentially suicidal behavior is essential, too:

:• Changes in personality

:• Failure to maintain personal hygiene

:• Lack of interest in activities

:• Running away from home

:• Depression

:• Sudden decline in school performance

:• Changes in appetite or sleep patterns

:• Extreme violent or aggressive behavior

:• Preoccupation with death and dying

:• Giving away possessions

:• Any suicide attempt, no matter how large or small

It would be remiss and irresponsible of us to not mention the fact that the most common method of suicide among young people is firearms. If any of your family members owns a gun, it is extremely important to take proper precautions with it, including trigger locks and locked cabinets. But this isn't just about guns, as the same precautions apply when family members have prescription medications at home that could lead to an overdose. You need to know what is in your home, because the likelihood is that your children probably know even more than you do.

4

Eating and Body Image

WHEN YOU HAVE been the one making decisions for your kids about, well, just about everything during elementary school, it can be jarring when suddenly these same sweet children assert more authority and independence in everything they do, from what they wear to whom they hang out with. And the fact is, our child's body is figuring out what it is supposed to look like—what shape it is supposed to take and what works best for it. What a tumultuous time for them—so they experiment with clothes, they feel good about themselves, they compare themselves with others, they get body-related messages from their peers, they feel terrible about themselves. And, of course, they are also getting the message from the media and popular culture that only one body type is "acceptable," while learning at the same time that the United States is experiencing an obesity crisis. What are they to think?

While we want to instill positive self-image and healthy habits in our children, we need to remember that eating—what to eat, and how much or how little—is one thing our adolescents can still control outright. Parents are thus in a precarious position when it comes to promoting good eating habits in children. On the one hand, we want to encourage them to make good dietary choices. On the other hand, if we focus too heavily on weight gain in our children, we may trigger unhealthy habits, hurt their feelings, or damage their sense of self.

On top of that, let's be honest: Parents send lots of mixed messages. All of us have complained about our own bodies at some point in front of our children; many of us still dread our own mothers' subtle or not-so-subtle comments while we're shopping for, say, bathing suits. We can't want that for this generation. We should want to do better.

Still, we have spoken to many parents who just aren't sure how to address dieting/weight gain, nutrition, and body image in their children. How do you know if your child has a problem in these areas? Are changes in their diet or body just part of adolescence or signs of a clinical eating disorder? We want to help you spot the red flags of disordered eating, whether it takes the form of overeating, food deprivation, or bulimia. We also want to point you in the right direction if it turns out that your child needs to seek help from a health care professional.

As you've probably figured out by now, we are equal opportunists. You should know that body concerns are not limited to females. We often assume that boys are immune to the pressures surrounding body image and diet, but studies reveal that teenage boys are vulnerable during this time period, too—whether they focus on bodybuilding, losing or gaining weight, or self-esteem issues—so we need to make sure that we pay attention to how boys feel about their bodies as well.

A study conducted by the Association of Teachers and Lecturers in England revealed that more than half of teachers noticed that the boys in their classrooms were obsessed with their body image and many had low self-confidence about their physical appearance. The report also showed that both boys and girls as young as four were worried about getting too fat. One teacher noted a kindergartener's remark at snack time: "I can't eat cheese—it will make me fat." In addition, the survey indicated that teachers witnessed girls discussing their feelings about body image more readily than boys did, but the boys, when asked directly, confessed their feelings, too.

Logan has taught hundreds of classes on sexual development and puberty. When she says that weight gain is a part of growing up, nearly everyone winces, even though she tells her students, "Gaining weight is not the same as becoming fat." We need our boys and girls to know that we are not all supposed to be skinny. In addition to being boring, in many cases it is downright unhealthy.

Yet there is tremendous pressure on both girls and boys to look like the images that the media bombards them with on a daily basis. The hairstyles, bodies, clothing, and makeup of pop stars, actors, and athletes are often popular among tweens and teens, yet pop culture's representation of the ideal body today is severely limited. Young people already have enough on their plates from academic and social pressure; adding body-image woes to the list can amp up the stress. Externally measuring themselves not only with their peers, but with airbrushed celebrities in the media as well, can lead to dangerous levels of pressure and disappointment.

1 My daughter just asked me if I think she's fat! She's a little overweight, but I don't want to hurt her feelings. What should I do?

Is this a damned-if-you-do, damned-if-you-don't question or what? There is a fine line between instilling a positive self-image in your child and creating a lifetime of self-loathing. In some ways, discussions about body image and weight can be the most difficult of all parent-child conversations. At least, that's how they feel to us. Give us a conversation about sex anytime!

Sadly, you are not the first parent whose child has asked this, and you certainly won't be the last. We can't tell you how many parents we have heard from—parents of fourth-, fifth-, even *first-graders*—who have gotten this same question from their kids. More often than not, the mothers are horrified that this behavior starts so young, but if you look at the media images that these kids are subjected to on a daily basis and some of the talk that they are probably overhearing from their parents, older siblings, or classmates, it's not really surprising.

A 1991 study from the National Eating Disorders Association revealed that 42 percent (that's more than four in ten) of kids in first through third grade wished they were thinner. Understandably, some parents are at a loss for how to deal with this issue, because most didn't experience this phenomenon when they were children. We feel, both as parents and as educators, that instilling positive body image in our children is one of the greatest challenges for parents today.

This whole issue makes us sad and angry. Quite frankly, we think it's bullshit that "I'm fat" has become a thing to say because our kids have heard others say it. It's bullshit that our children are bonding over self-loathing and body hatred. We've become a society that expects people to reject their own bodies while feeding them airbrushed images to digest like M&M's. It's not okay, it is certainly not productive, and it should all stop here!

We can start by trying to figure out where this sentiment is coming from, because it may not be what you expect. Sometimes girls and boys express body hatred when what they are really trying to express is fear and anxiety over the physical changes that occur during puberty. Engaging in a dialogue with your child may make this approach more apparent. It's also important not to dismiss their feelings by saying, "Oh, don't be ridiculous—you're not fat" and then just leaving it at that. When you hear your child express this kind of talk, a conversation is in order. We need to take the time to listen to what our children are saying, even if the comments seem to be misguided or irrational. Your child may need to vent; we need to listen and then reinforce how we all need to be less judgmental of ourselves and more accepting of our individuality.

Don't freak out if your child insists on dieting; just be sure to emphasize healthful habits, rather than weight. You can encourage regular exercise, wise food choices, good sleep habits, and stress relief as part of an overall plan. Studies show that incorporating this approach early on in life paves the way for better habits later in life.

And don't forget to model good behavior. If you ever say that you want to lose weight in front of your child or ask if you look fat in something, you need to stop doing it. And please don't think that we are perfect in this department, but when we find ourselves misstepping, we quickly turn it around. We are human, too, and part of being human means that we need to constantly monitor our own behaviors and conversations. Even from a young age, kids are sponges. As their parent, you are a powerful role model, probably more than you realize. We need to do a better job at keeping those negative comments to ourselves or, better yet, try to eliminate them from our psyches. Yes, it's easier said than done, but the change in attitude needs to start with us.

2 My son is definitely overweight but doesn't seem to care. Should I?

Should you care? Well, yes, but for the right reasons. You should care because being overweight can lead to other health issues. You should care because he may not even realize that he's overweight. His lack of noticing (or caring) in some ways may be a positive thing (he has good self-esteem and his peers don't make an issue of his weight), or it may be that he has so detached himself from his body that he's sort of checked out. Weight gain and loss is hard enough to manage for adults; for teens, it's even more challenging.

Having said that, we do not believe in fat shaming. We don't believe in shaming of any variety, in fact. We want our children to be healthy, and skinny is not synonymous with healthy. Research published in 2013 in the scientific journal of the Public Library of Science revealed that shaming people about their weight doesn't help them lose weight; in fact, it may have the opposite effect. We need to make it clear to our children that our concern is about their health, not their looks. (We know that you may secretly be concerned about their appearance as well, but your children *definitely* do not need to know this.)

Nonetheless, this a conversation that needs to be broached delicately. It shouldn't take place in front of other people (like embarrassing a child at dinner in front of family, friends, and so on). When you have a quiet moment with your child, try saying something like this: "I want to talk to you about something. I love you so much, and I want you to have every opportunity in life. I want you to be healthy, and I'm afraid that your eating habits and/or lack of exercise are hindering you. What do you think we can do to help you to be as healthy as possible?"

But you should know that the situation you find yourself in is not uncommon. The number of overweight kids in the United

States is increasing at an alarming rate. According to the Office of the Surgeon General, one in three kids in the United States is either overweight or at risk of becoming overweight.

Many children are spending less time exercising and more time in front of electronic media, from televisions to computers to iPads. Other reports reveal that more and more families are opting for quick-and-easy meals, which may be loaded with calories, and fewer sit-down, communal dinners. Busy schedules make this the new reality for many families. And don't think we're judging you—we're managing these issues in our own lives too.

The challenge lies in encouraging our children to adopt a healthy lifestyle, and that begins with the parents. It's very important to pay attention to the way your family eats and exercises and how you spend time together. Your own food choices and exercise routines are models for your kids. So if you skip off to spin class on Saturday morning or go for a power walk or a run, your children get the message that exercise is a priority. And if you keep healthful snacks—like vegetables, fruits, and nuts—in the house, rather than chips and cookies, you instill better nutritional values in your kids.

This isn't a superficial conversation. Being overweight increases the risk of all sorts of health issues for children. And even though you will love your son no matter what weight he is, you want him to be as healthy as possible. For this reason, when you discuss this subject with him, focus on the health aspects of being overweight, including risk of high blood pressure, diabetes, asthma, sleep disturbances, social issues, and depression. For girls, being overweight can present its own set of issues, such as early puberty and menstrual irregularities. And both male and female overweight children and adolescents are much more likely to become overweight adults with unhealthy diets and sedentary lifestyles, which are known risk factors for cancer, heart disease, and stroke later in life. So breaking bad habits and encouraging good ones early on can have major benefits down the road. There really is no time like the present to start making positive lifestyle changes.

Ultimately, the way your son takes care of his body is his decision. Constantly focusing on his weight may backfire and make him feel embarrassed and self-conscious. You want to empower him, not make him miserable, but sometimes finding that balance can be difficult. Enlist the help of a health care professional. Speak to his doctor ahead of time, and during your son's next visit, ask the doctor to bring up the importance of healthy eating habits and daily exercise. Discuss the concept of body mass index (BMI), and make a plan together to focus on healthy living. Hearing this information from non–family members, especially health care workers, may mean it makes an especially lasting impression on your son.

❸ My daughter exercises every day, and I'm a little worried. How do I know if it's too much?

Exercise is obviously much better than sitting around all day in front of a computer, munching on Fritos, but your concern may not be out of line. There's a point at which exercising can become unhealthy; the tricky part is recognizing when it becomes too much of a good thing.

The term *compulsive exercise* describes behavior that takes exercise to an excessive level on a daily basis. People who are compulsive exercisers work out so much that they place themselves at risk of physical and emotional injury. Their rigorous routines can wear down their body, increase their potential for injury, and damage their emotional well-being. The behavior is a lot like an eating disorder and can become just as addictive.

Compulsive exercise can affect both girls and boys, though it seems to be most common in girls and in people of either gender who participate in organized athletics. Sports that focus on weight and/or physical appearance, including ballet, gymnastics, wrestling, swimming, track and field, crew, and cheerleading—many of the same sports liable to promote eating disorders—are particularly prone to creating compulsive exercisers, too.

Studies show that more than 90 percent of women who have bulimia nervosa (binge eating with purging) exercise to compensate for bingeing. Girls and boys who have eating disorders are at higher risk of becoming preoccupied with exercise.

Exercise is great, but it's important to know when it's become a problem for our children. Here are some of the things to look for:

- Working out several times a day

- Exercising despite an injury

:• Changing habits to accommodate exercise (skipping meals, skimping on sleep, letting grades slip)

:• Exercising in bad weather (rain, snow, hurricanes!)

:• Preoccupation with exercise (talking about it all the time, etc.)

If you think your child is exercising compulsively, we highly recommend addressing the issue. Oftentimes an underlying cause triggers this type of behavior. Examples include pressure from a coach, teammates, or parents; strong emotions that need an outlet; weight loss; or an attempt to regain a feeling of control over one aspect of one's life.

Overexercising can cause real health consequences, including wear-and-tear injuries like shin splints, stress fractures, and damage to muscles and joints. Compulsive exercisers frequently "push through the pain" or exercise while injured, so their injuries rarely have a chance to heal. For girls, extreme exercising and weight loss can cause amenorrhea, or loss of their monthly menstrual cycle. Prolonged amenorrhea can increase their risk of brittle bones, heart problems, and fertility issues later in life.

If you think your daughter's behavior can be characterized as compulsive exercise, she needs to get help. Treatment varies bases on each case but may involve a doctor (especially if she has any physical injuries), a therapist (who can address any underlying emotional issues), and/or a nutritionist (especially if your daughter has disordered eating habits as well).

4 Many of my girlfriends are juicing or doing a periodic juice cleanse. My fourteen-year-old just asked if he could juice, too.

There are definitely some things you should take into consideration when discussing this subject with your son. If he isn't big on fruits and vegetables, juicing can be a great way to incorporate these foods into his diet, as one eight-ounce glass of juice is often packed with a ton of vitamins and nutrients. But it shouldn't be his only source of fruits and vegetables; the juicing machine removes all of the pulp, which contains fiber, so he's missing out on that and needs to get it from other sources. The skin, which is full of benefits, also gets separated, so it's important to eat whole fruits and vegetables, as well as bran.

Juice cleansing is another story. Claims that a juice cleanse can "detox" or cleanse your body of toxins lack scientific support and data. The body is equipped to do this on its own through an elaborate digestive system involving your liver and kidney. Consuming only juice for several days at a time can be unhealthy, so we do not recommend it as a proper dietary choice for children and adolescents. Many people end up consuming far too few calories and feel light-headed, dizzy, and undernourished or have headaches and stomachaches. It is too important for growing bodies to have a properly balanced diet, filled with all of the food groups, on a daily basis.

Besides, eating real food is enjoyable. Logan attempted a three-day juice cleanse a few years ago. Here's what she says about the experience:

I love to eat. The only things I drink are coffee, margaritas, wine, and water (if I have to). But my girlfriends and I were going to try this highly publicized cleanse together. The first day was torture. I had a dull headache that wouldn't go away, and I was nasty to be around. By the second morning, I gave up. I was hungry and missed chewing food. I was completely unsatisfied. In addition to being a total waste of money, it made me miserable. Nothing was worth that. My children and my husband couldn't bear to be around me—and I only juiced for twenty-four hours. Imagine if I had gone through the full three days!

The celebrity-cleanse craze is problematic for all of us. Most adults and children do not live the lives of celebrities. Most of us do not have trainers, nutritionists, surgeons, makeup artists, and personal assistants to cater to our every whim. While a cleanse may "work" for those people (though we remain unconvinced that it does), developing bodies need nutritious food, not "cleansing."

5 My daughter thinks her best friend is anorexic and wants to help. I'm not sure how to guide her.

We commend your daughter for being a concerned and caring friend. Anorexia nervosa is an eating disorder that involves an extreme fear of gaining weight or being fat. It affects girls more often than boys and often involves a distorted body image—that is, many people see themselves as fat even though they are very thin.

Anorexia nervosa is a serious condition that needs to be addressed, diagnosed, and treated by medical professionals. Warning signs include the following:

:• Consistent food deprivation

:• Extreme fear of gaining weight

:• Looking much thinner (this can occur over time or in a short period)

:• Excessive monitoring of weight (e.g., always stepping on a scale)

:• Wearing big, baggy clothes to hide the body

:• Avoiding mealtime (for example, a person walks around the cafeteria during lunch instead of sitting down to eat with friends)

As anorexia nervosa progresses, some of the following physical signs may become apparent:

:• Mood swings and irritability

:• Difficulty concentrating

:• Bruising

:• Thermoregulation, or a person's internal temperature regulation, becomes faulty (the person gets cold very easily)

:• Hair thinning or loss

:• Fine hair grows on face or body

:• For girls, menstrual periods become irregular or stop altogether (this is known as amenorrhea)

If your daughter's friend is anorexic, one of the best things
she can do is to encourage her friend to seek help. This can be
a very challenging proposition, because many people who suffer
from eating disorders fully deny that they have a problem. Your
daughter can also try to approach her friend's parents and voice
her concern. Sometimes girls who suffer from eating issues have
mothers, sisters, or close relatives who have also battled an eating
disorder. This is definitely something to keep in mind, no matter
who brings up the issue with your daughter's friend.

**6 I've been trying to lose weight lately and have tried
many different diets. I recently found one that works
for me, and now my daughter wants to go on it. Should
I let her?**

No. How's that for simplicity? You're a grown-up; she isn't. And
while we're on the subject, let's talk a little bit about the danger of
fad diets for both you and your daughter. "Miracle" diet plans are
everywhere, many filled with promises of immediate weight loss

within a few days or even overnight. These diets have wide appeal, and why wouldn't they? Everyone loves a quick fix. The problem is that many of these diets are unhealthy and the results, if there are any, are usually short-lived. Many studies reveal that people on fad diets regain much of the weight within two to three months after coming off the diet.

Depriving the body of food from a wide variety of food groups can cause real health consequences. So many fad diets eliminate major food groups—for example, carbohydrates, milk and dairy products, or meat—and therefore cause headaches, dizziness, fatigue, low blood sugar, and nausea, among other conditions. Aside from these numerous health problems, growing children have unique health and dietary requirements that shouldn't be ignored. Growing tweens and teenagers need calcium and vitamin D. If the diet your daughter wants to try involves eliminating dairy and milk products at this crucial stage in her development, she is putting herself at risk for osteoporosis, a condition characterized by brittle bones and loss of bone mass, that some pediatricians are seeing signs of in teens and young women. A study at Bristol University in England that used scanning devices to calculate the shape and density of the bones of four thousand fifteen year olds revealed that teenage girls who frequently diet are at higher risk for osteoporosis.

And these health concerns don't pertain only to your daughter—parents need to be aware of the risks for themselves, too. Our recommendation is to avoid anything that promises rapid weight loss over a short period of time, tells you to avoid certain food groups, or promotes only one type of food. Eating grapefruits all day for a week gets old pretty quickly, and the negative side effects this type of behavior can induce far outweigh any short-term weight-loss benefits for you and especially for your daughter.

7 I just found out from one of the moms at school that my daughter is throwing up between classes. I'm distraught. How can I help her?

It's okay to be distraught—your daughter needs medical attention. Getting her the resources and help she needs should be your first priority.

Now that we've been up front about that, we need to better understand what this particular type of behavior is all about. It will not only help you to get a better sense of what your daughter might be going through but also serve as a mirror for you and some of the issues that we inadvertently bring to our children's attention.

Bulimia nervosa is characterized by eating a substantial amount of food (bingeing) and then clearing the body of the calories by throwing up or using laxatives and/or diuretics (purging). Bulimics may also fast for twenty-four hours after a purge or engage in excessive bouts of exercise to cancel out the calories. Bulimics frequently report that they have difficulty controlling their eating behavior, and that they use food as a comfort and then purge or restrict for relief. Many people who suffer from bulimia have body-image issues.

Recent studies have shown an alarming rise in eating disorders among children. The Agency for Healthcare Research and Quality revealed that hospitalizations for eating disorders in children under the age of twelve increased by 119 percent between 1999 and 2006. While 2013 figures aren't yet available, many experts claim that the problem is only getting worse.

Spotting the signs of bulimia nervosa can be challenging for a parent, especially because many bulimics try to conceal their behavior. A few mothers have asked up if throwing up just a few times constitutes bulimia. The take-home message is that throwing up your food on purpose is never healthy, but to be formally diagnosed with bulimia nervosa, a person needs to have two binge-purge cycles per week for at least three months. Bingeing and purging is a hard cycle to break; many patients report having little control over their behavior after initially feeling like it was no big deal and they could stop whenever they wanted.

The following are some behavioral signs to look for in your child:

:• Secrecy surrounding eating (going to the kitchen after everyone else is sleeping; wanting to eat in private)

:• Disappearance of food (empty wrappers, stashing junk food, etc.)

:• Eating significant amounts of food (this may alternate with periods of fasting)

:• Going to the bathroom after/during meals (many kids run the sink faucet to hide the sounds of their vomiting)

:• Smell of vomit in the bathroom (some try to conceal it with deodorizers, mouthwash, etc.)

:• Excessive exercise after meals

The following are some physical signs to pay attention to in your child:

:• Swollen cheeks caused by repetitive vomiting

:• Redness, cuts, or calluses on knuckles from sticking fingers down the throat to trigger vomiting

:• Erosion of tooth enamel from stomach acid during vomiting episodes

:• Irregular bowel movements; constipation from chronic laxative abuse

:• Swelling of parotid and/or salivary glands

Now, the tricky thing about bulimia is that bulimics may not be underweight. They are often normal weight or even slightly overweight, and they are not just girls. Hear that? Eating disorders of all kinds can affect all people, regardless of gender. Recent studies show that the numbers of boys affected may be higher than most people realize. The number of male binge eaters ranges from 10 to 40 percent, which isn't the common representation of someone suffering from an eating disorder.

It can be incredibly unnerving for a parent whose child is suffering from an eating disorder. But because it's such a serious issue, you must approach your child. We know that it is easier said than done, but try to bring up the topic in a calm, caring, and nonjudgmental way. Tell your child what you heard from other parents or classmates, express your love and concern, and try to listen—kids with eating disorders may be afraid, embarrassed, or in denial. Some will downplay their behavior, in which case you'll have to revisit the topic several times. Be persistent, and always let them know you want to help.

The Internet provides parents with some amazing insights into children's behaviors. Pay attention to what your kids are viewing. Many horrifying pro–eating disorder websites exist, and YouTube has some videos that promote eating disorders. There are some immediate clues: these sites often use the phrases *pro-ana* (for anorexia) and *pro-mia* (for bulimia). If technology is being used under your roof (and you are paying for it), you have a right to see what it is being used for.

8 **Every time my daughter looks at fashion magazines, she complains about her body. This can't be healthy. Should I take them away?**

The short answer is no, though we'd like to say yes. Hiding magazines from your children isn't going to solve our cultural problem of unhealthy images and the lack of diversity represented in our media. However, you are right to be concerned. Tweens and teenage girls are bombarded with images of female models, celebrities, and rock stars in magazines, on television shows, and online on a daily basis. Many experts have debated how this media storm has an impact on the psyche of adolescents, especially girls. According to data from the NYU Child Study Center, among fifth- to twelfth-grade girls, 47 percent said that they wanted to lose weight because of the photos they saw in magazines. Among the same age group, 60 percent of girls were dissatisfied with their body shape.

In 2012, Jena's oldest daughter started collecting tween magazines that showcased her favorite singer, Taylor Swift; her room is lined with cutouts and posters. Jena knows that banning the images wouldn't make her daughter like those magazines any less. Instead, she uses them as a means of talking about Taylor Swift's (or any other teen idol's) accomplishments. If and when the conversation strays into what these stars are wearing and what they look like, Jena tries to steer it in another direction, one that emphasizes hard work and talent.

To complicate matters, brands strategically place their magazine advertisements in order to dictate what their readers should
aspire to look like, purchase, and wear. According to the American
Psychology Association, more than one in five girls read teen magazines for at least twenty minutes per day. No matter where you
live, girls (especially those in the early teenage years) want to fit in;
it is developmentally appropriate for them, and means they want
to—they *need* to—wear the latest trends.

Don't believe us? Eighty percent of girls have purchased an
item as a result of seeing an ad in a teen magazine; 63 percent trust
magazine ads. (Logan admits that while she doesn't always buy
things she sees in ads, she will go online to check them out.) In a
society that emphasizes materialism, it shouldn't be a surprise that
girls are easily convinced that they require particular fashions to
belong.

It's also not surprising that this perspective can affect their
self-esteem. Some experts believe that these images can have a
damaging and lasting effect on girls' sense of self. Being hit over
the head with images of ideal beauty and body types can leave
anyone—let alone girls going through the significant developmental stage that puberty represents—feeling as if they can never
measure up. And despite the fact that many kids realize these
images have been airbrushed or touched up, they still feel the
pressure to conform.

They are not alone—celebrities feel the pressure, too. Christina
Aguilera, singer and judge on *The Voice*, has been the victim of

brutal media criticism bordering on verbal assault for gaining weight. Jena was driving a carpool and overheard the girls in the back discussing the issue. Jena's daughter asked her friends, "Why does it matter what she weighs? Does she claim to be world's skinniest person, or is she a singer? Does she work with her voice or her body?" When silence took over the backseat and no one had a good answer to that question, the conversation shifted to how talented a singer Christina Aguilera is. We need to teach our young people to be better critical thinkers in all aspects of their life.

But our point is this: Girls are *grossly* misrepresented in our media. They are sexualized and in turn taught that their value is based solely on their looks—specifically on their bodies. It is no wonder that our girls (and boys for that matter, too) buy into what they see; they don't see anything different. Thin torsos, sculpted abdominal muscles, large breasts, and thigh gaps have all become desirable, media-generated physical traits.

We need to provide diversity for our children. We need to show them how conventional definitions of beauty evolve over time and how cultures have different standards for what they consider beautiful. Show your children art that is representative of different body shapes, and teach them to be critical of the images that keep showing up. There are some positive developments arising in this area, such as the Dove Campaign for Real Beauty, which is designed to combat unrealistic images of beauty; however, even this concept isn't without controversy, as critics have complained that Dove's message can be misconstrued as counterintuitive.

Perhaps the most poignant take on how girls are represented in pop culture comes from the 2012 documentary *Miss
Representation*. Watch it and see how pervasive these unhealthy
images are. You may want to show your children parts of the film.
Give them the tools to stand up and fight for diversity and respect
in the media. If we don't teach them to do it, no one will.

**⑨ All of the guys on my son's football team are trying to
gain weight, but my son doesn't want to eat huge portions
of food like his friends do. He's worried he'll be much
smaller than the team. How can I advise him?**

We have already mentioned some of the sports that encourage
food restriction, which can place athletes at higher risk of developing eating disorders. But there are also sports in which athletes are
urged to gain mass to improve their performance. This behavior is
sometimes seen on football teams and, if not adopted properly, can
have health consequences.

Eating for the sole purpose of rapidly gaining weight can be
dangerous. Some of the risks include skin problems, muscle and
joint injuries, high blood pressure, and diabetes. Another issue for parents to consider is the use of supplements to increase
muscle mass and body size. Oftentimes adolescent athletes ignore
the label's recommendations and overdose on these supplements,
which can cause electrolyte imbalances and kidney stones and can

increase the potential for vitamin toxicity. Many of these supplements aren't regulated by the FDA, and the products' claims may be inaccurate and invalid.

So in this case, your son's instincts are right. Gaining weight is not always synonymous with being stronger. And who wants to act like a competitive eater just to fit in? In fact, athletic skill isn't limited to what someone's body looks like; it depends upon the sport. If your son is a linebacker, sure, size counts. But if he's a quarterback or a receiver, he needs to be quick on his feet.

Our recommendation is to commend your son for having the courage to trust his instincts. The staff working with the football team should be made aware of the situation. There are safe ways to increase muscle mass, but the athletes should be under the guidance of adults who can encourage and oversee healthy diet, exercise, and strength training/weightlifting programs.

10 My son is overweight and recently asked me if he's going to die young because he's obese. Help!

Death and obesity do seem to be linked. At least, that's what our media suggests. No matter how we try to shield our children from mainstream news, they get the message: Obesity can be fatal. So tread lightly, because while you don't want to scare your son, the facts are the facts.

However, it is important to recognize that there is something good about this scenario. Your son is aware that his health may be impacted by his weight. Parents who are unsure whether their children are obese often approach us for advice about how they can help their children. The first step is to recognize that there's a problem, and it seems that your son is already aware he may need to lose weight. For many people, that's the biggest battle.

Overweight and *obese* are both labels for weight ranges greater than what is generally considered healthy for a given height, according to the Centers for Disease Control and Prevention. The terms also identify weight ranges that have been shown to increase the risk of certain health problems and diseases.

Schools across the United States have implemented programs to combat childhood obesity, within both cafeterias and physical-education curricula. Michelle Obama's Let's Move! initiative and Jamie Oliver's Food Revolution are just two examples of how schools (with the help of parents and community leaders) effect behavioral changes.

Chances are, your son has probably heard much about obesity from a variety of sources. One of the negative things about this scenario is that it sounds like he is frightened, and he shouldn't be. Instead, as his parent, you can empower him to take charge of his own health and to make the necessary lifestyle and nutritional changes to bring his weight into a healthy range.

Remember, boys and girls develop at different rates, so it isn't always easy to know if your child is overweight or obese. We recommend checking in with your health care provider and requesting that your son's height and weight be measured, to determine whether he is in a healthy range for his age. If the doctor determines that your child needs a weight-loss program, we recommend involving the entire family so he doesn't feel singled out. Adding more fruits and vegetables to his diet and limiting juices, soda, and high-calorie snacks can help, as can daily physical activity. The US Department of Health and Human Services and the National Institutes of Health recommend sixty minutes of physical activity per day for children who are dealing with weight issues.

Thankfully, exercise doesn't have to be boring or traditional these days. Your son has lots of options. Even if he doesn't love athletics, he can think outside of the box: martial arts, boxing, hiking, fencing, rock climbing, weight lifting, or rowing are all possibilities. If he is uncomfortable with the idea of competitive sports, encourage a life sport, such as running or cycling, that can build up his endurance. If he likes the idea of team sports, look for one grouped by skill level. Some evidence suggests that overweight teens may benefit from joining a sports team that is organized by skill instead of by age.

⑪ My daughter is on a diet, and I overheard her telling her friend that the boys will finally like her if she loses ten pounds and wears short skirts. How should I address this?

This question makes our hearts hurt, because both of us, at some point or another, have felt the same way. We can remember a time when we thought our bodies were what made us attractive to someone else. Of course, while that was a long time ago, our world is chock-full of messaging and imagery that make all of our children (regardless of gender) buy into the notion that their worth is measured by their bodies and not their brains.

What we need to be doing is asking our children to think about what makes someone likable. Is it hair? Muscles? Breast size? Is it how much money that person has? Our children need to understand that superficial qualities do not guarantee a good relationship and certainly don't mean that people will respect you or treat you well.

But we're not about to stick our heads in the sand. We do understand how powerful the urge to fit in, to be perceived as beautiful, even sexy, is. So what can we do about it? We can show our children how those standards vary from person to person and culture to culture. We can show our children what we wear when we want to feel most beautiful. It may be a suit; it may be pajamas. Chances are, it won't be a skintight skirt or a revealing top. But if it is, consider this: Sometimes we like ourselves in clingy clothes because we have worked hard to take care of our bodies. We feel good about the skin we're in, but not because someone else likes us better that way. Therein lies the difference.

So how do you bring this up? Delicately, but you have to do it. And it's not just about you—it should also be a conversation that your male parenting partner (if you have one) has with your daughter. Men need to model for their children how men should treat women, and vice versa. Women should be doing the same for their sons. It's about respect.

Try a version of this: "Honey, we want to talk to you about something we overheard. We weren't eavesdropping, but we heard you say that boys would like you if you lost weight and dressed differently. People shouldn't like you because of how you look; they should like you because of who you are. Someone who respects you doesn't want you to change; he should make you feel comfortable and loved in your own skin. I understand that you want to fit in, but changing for someone else will never make you happy in the end. If you're not happy now, what can we do to help you?"

Validating your daughter's feelings is essential. It is far easier to belittle them than it is to hear that she may be hurting, but what she needs is for you to be a sounding board and a source of support.

5

Social Media and Technology

I N CASE YOU'VE been living in a world without newspapers, magazines, or the eleven o'clock news, sexting is the act of sending sexually explicit messages or pictures between mobile devices, such as iPods, cell phones, and tablets. In 2011 and 2012, a few cases of sexting made front-page headlines, creating a media frenzy that sparked a series of nationwide, school-sponsored attempts to alert teens to the dangers of sexting, as well as some less rational law-enforcement efforts to prosecute teens as sex offenders and for possessing and distributing child pornography.

However, several studies, including one published in December 2011 in the journal *Pediatrics*, reveal that sexting is not as common as many parents may think. According to this study, roughly one in one hundred teens has personally engaged in sexting, though media outlets originally estimated this number to be as high as one in five. (You see, we told you there are lots of alarmist headlines out there!) Out of that group that *Pediatrics* surveyed, only 10 percent of the kids who took images actually distributed them, and just 3 percent who received them forwarded the pictures to others.

While the statistics are in our favor, the fact that sexting exists and has led to legal proceedings (and severe consequences) means that we shouldn't take this topic lightly and should discuss it with our children. Using technology respectfully is an essential part of today's adolescence. And here's the thing: Is it any surprise that our kids are using technology to express their sexuality? Definitely not. (We were doing it on those chat lines in the late '80s and early '90s, and we said some horrible things there—things that we would be mortified to have attributed to us today.) The difference was that at that time there was anonymity and no permanent digital trail. So it is our job to understand why kids do this and, more importantly, to teach them how to best express themselves using social media and technology—and this is as much a conversation about friendship as it is about dating and sex.

We know that the combination of kids and technology makes parents especially nervous, in no small part because many teens are more digitally savvy than we are. Since technology is evolving so rapidly, it is very important to establish an open dialogue about texting, social media, and proper use of cell phones from an early age (after all, even a two year old can scroll through an iPad and open the YouTube app—we know this personally).

The issues we find parents struggling with most often are how to simply keep up with trends, when and if to give kids a cell phone, what video games are appropriate, and how to properly monitor children's activities. Many parents we spoke with joined Facebook, for example, only to find that their kids had found other social-media networks to engage in that were seemingly parent-free. As we've mentioned before, the landscape of social media and digital technology is constantly changing. Just when you thought you've heard the ultimate stupid online trend, something even more ridiculous pops up. For us, though, the message is always the same, no matter what new gimmick comes our way.

1 I've been considering getting my child a cell phone, but she's begging me for a smartphone. Is she old enough?

Why do you want your daughter to have a cell phone? Do you want to be able to contact her? Do you want her to have a phone in case of emergency? Do you want her to text her friends at all hours of the night? (Okay, that wasn't a serious question, but you understand what we're getting at.) If a smartphone meets your needs for your child, then by all means get it for her, but not without checking out the other options available to you, too.

We worry that in an effort to be "cool," we have collectively forgotten how to parent. This issue comes up over and over again among our friends, peers, and colleagues. Perhaps more significantly, we've lived it. Jena's teenage daughter has a cell phone, but not an iPhone, and has been asking for an iPhone almost every day for an entire year. Jena has heard every justification under the sun, from "Everyone has one" to "I need it for school" to "You don't want me to be the only one without one, do you?"

Most parents aren't immune to this kind of badgering. Even as she writes this book, Jena wonders, *Am I turning my daughter into a loser?* But then she comes to her senses. Not only is a smartphone simply not necessary at this stage, but in fact, as Instagram, FaceTime, Snapchat, and Vine take over the social lives of her daughter's peers, Jena thinks her daughter is actually better off without one for now.

This doesn't mean that you categorically shouldn't give your child one of those super-jazzed-up mini-computer cell phones. But first, ask yourself these questions: Does she need it? And does she deserve it? Maybe you have the kind of kid who is thoughtful and responsible and generous with her friends and family. Maybe she makes good decisions and is quick to challenge her friends when they don't. Maybe she can use this smartphone in a "smart" way and not be distracted by it. Or maybe she can't. The fact is, even adults have a hard time focusing on the world in front of them while their phones are buzzing away. And we know better.

Regardless of the age your child is when you deem her ready for a smartphone, consider giving her a clear, written list of rules for using it—a contract of sorts. You can always have her sign it to make it even more formal. That puts responsibility into your daughter's hands; if she wants maturity and independence, she's going to have to prove she's ready.

The following is a sample contract:

Having a smartphone is a responsibility, and one that should not be taken lightly. I agree to the following rules:

I will not take pictures of myself or my friends without our clothes on.

I will not take pictures of myself or my friends doing anything that would get me (or them) in trouble.

I will not forward any questionable pictures that I may receive to anyone else.

My parent has the right to check my phone at any time for any reason.

I may not use my phone to write mean or nasty things about my friends or peers.

I will not use my phone after 9:00 PM without permission. [If this part is confusing to you, check the part of this book on sleep-related questions in chapters 1 and 3.]

I will not use my phone at the dinner table or other family gatherings.

I will charge my phone outside my bedroom and leave it there overnight.

This whole exercise may sound silly to you. But the point of it is to show you that kids and teens need explicit rules when it comes to using digital technology. They may know these rules already, but you still need to be clear. And there *must* be consequences if they breach this contract. They will never learn anything unless you hold them accountable.

2 **My son basically texts all the time. I asked him about it, and he said, "Why do I need to actually, like, talk to someone when I can just text them?" Help!**

It is our responsibility to teach our children what it means to be a fully functioning human being. Part of this effort includes knowing how to communicate with people—more specifically, knowing how to communicate with people face-to-face.

Your own habits play a big role in this regard. Jena was at the library one day, reading to her toddler, when an older boy came and sat down next to them. They read together for a little while, until the older boy got up to look for his mom. When he couldn't find her, he became startled and ran around the library. His mom was texting in the back of the children's library, without a clue that her son had wandered off. When Jena let the mother know that her son was upset, the woman couldn't even be bothered to look up from her cell phone.

All of the advancements in communication since we were children don't eliminate the need for personal contact. As parents, we're the ones who need to instill these skills in our children. To work toward this goal, you can encourage your child to:

- Listen attentively

- Maintain eye contact

- Not interrupt the person speaking, and ask questions only when that person is finished

- Use body language to convey that they are engaged, and maintain proper posture

- Speak clearly, enunciate, and use proper tone of voice, i.e., not be snappy, snarky, overly sarcastic, or rude

Common sense, right? We used to think so, but we can't tell you how many parents have asked us for these tips. We are increasingly concerned that the art of interpersonal, nonelectronic communication is getting lost, even among babysitters and summer counselors and parents of all ages. One night while we were writing this book, Jena sat next to a family of four at a restaurant. The kids were probably around nine and twelve years old. The family did not exchange a single word as each person at the table texted, looked at their phone screen, and barely glanced up at the waiter to order.

Language comes in many forms. However, what makes texting particularly challenging is that it involves a loss of both body language and tone of voice. We don't care how many smiley faces pepper the screen—the writer could be flipping off your child simultaneously. There is no way to verify the intent of a text, so the recipient may take what is written out of context. While we all know texting is here to stay, face-to-face communication is a vital skill that your child will need to master for success in life.

3 My daughter's friends are calling her names on Facebook. Is this bullying? What should I do?

It's heart-wrenching for parents to hear that their child feels like they are being picked on. Bullying can take many forms, but the Internet allows for a more insidious type of bullying, because it allows for people to believe that they are less accountable for their actions.

Before you pick up the phone to call someone's parents, ask your daughter to show you what she is talking about. Bullying can sometimes feel different to different people, and one of the problems with online bullying is that the real meaning behind the written words can be difficult to assess, so people sometimes read too much into a comment. Here are a few things to consider:

:• Is the language threatening or intimidating?

:• Is the language mean-spirited or cruel?

:• Is there a pattern? Is your child actually being harassed, or is she simply the victim of an isolated, albeit thought-less, comment?

In this particular case, you are going to have to ask your child the following questions: What are these names that you're being called? Are other people getting in on it? (You will be devastated no matter what the answers are, but at least this will give you a sense of what is going on.) You are going to also need to ask your daughter if there is anything that may have provoked the name calling. We are not suggesting that you blame the victim, as name calling is never justified; on the contrary, we just want you to have all of the facts.

Once you do, you can call your daughter's friends' parents. Ask them if they have seen what their kids are posting online. This is not to encourage tattling but rather to say that we need to be more involved in our kids' online presence.

While talking to parents is important, you also want to em-power your child. We need to encourage teenage girls to take ownership of their voice. For example, has your daughter told the person or people who posted the offensive comments to stop? Sometimes a firm voice is all it takes; your daughter will feel like she has dealt with the comments on her own.

Handling this situation responsibly also means ending it re-spectfully. Discourage your child from writing back anything offensive. While it might feel good in the moment to dish it out, this kind of response typically escalates the situation and lets the people know that whatever they wrote is bothering your child.

If the name calling and online harassment don't stop, there are steps your daughter can take to protect herself. She can report the behavior and posts to Facebook, requesting that action be taken to remove the posts, especially if they are public; she can also close her account and open a new one when this blows over. In addition, parents can report on behalf of minors. Many social networking sites have guidelines for parents and caregivers.

If the situation continues to escalate, you may want to involve someone at your child's school. While a guidance counselor might not be able to handle the harassment directly, it could benefit your daughter to make someone at her school aware of the situation so they can check in with her as needed. Of course, if your daughter ever receives physical threats, racial taunts, or photos that are demeaning and/or involve nudity, you should notify the police immediately.

4 The majority of my son's friends play *Call of Duty* on the Xbox, but I really don't like those first-person shooter games. I won't let him play, but he told me that I'm turning him into a loser. Any advice?

As you know, we're realists. We know that the minute children leave the house, they might do all the things we have forbidden them to do in their own home. In other words, the chances that your son is playing *Call of Duty* at a friend's house are good. However, we also believe that the quantity and content of violence in popular video games are atrocious, and we would not want those games in our house either.

As parents, we might consider the following question: Is there a real connection between violent video games and violent behavior? Given that first-person shooter games represent a $5 billion market and are played by millions of people every day, it's a scary thought. After the Newtown, Connecticut, school shooting in December 2012, it was widely reported that the killer was an avid *Call of Duty* player. Was there a link? And do you need to worry about your son's own potential for violence if he plays violent video games?

When you look at the studies (though we admit there haven't been a ton), the answers are not so clear. Some researchers claim that first-person shooter games influence violent behavior. While there is not a direct cause-and-effect relationship, these games can make violence more likely to occur in vulnerable individuals. The tricky part of this idea is the fact that the concept of "vulnerability" is not yet well defined.

Other researchers argue that there is no link and that certain children are simply prone to violent acts, regardless of their access to video games. It's easy to become confused and unsure about whether these games are really harmful or not. Some parents simply feel unequipped (and sometimes just too emotionally exhausted) to engage in the fight with their children. One of Jena's close friends, who is also a doctor, grappled with this issue in her home when her ninth-grade son wanted to play a first-person shooter game that required him and his friends to connect to each other online, through headsets, as they sat in their respective homes. She was torn at first but eventually caved and even purchased the most recent edition as a birthday gift for her son. "What can I do?" she asked Jena. "Everyone else plays it."

So here's the challenge: We don't want our children to feel like they are "losers," but we don't want them to think that we are comfortable with simulated violence if we aren't. Logan is constantly horrified by the seemingly acceptable violence against women in video games (and on television). In her home, games that deliberately target women (whether they are prostitutes or not) are nonnegotiable. But it's really a judgment call on your part, and, as with everything else in life, you have to pick your battles. For us, this is one of them. For you, it may not be.

5 **The mom of my daughter's best friend just told me that my daughter sent some topless pictures to her boyfriend. I'm worried that her boyfriend could share the photos with other people, and I don't know how to address this with my daughter.**

Unfortunately, you need to handle this sooner rather than later, for all of the above reasons and more. First, we know that your initial response may be to want to strangle your daughter. How could she be so stupid? We hear you, but before you scream and yell, take a moment to think about what she's going through.

She's young, and she's trying to figure out how to appropriately express her feelings and her sexuality. As adults, we see this as complete and utter stupidity, but really, it's not that surprising. Young people are used to hearing the "just say no" message when it comes to sex. If you are a teenager, you are probably thinking, *Okay, my parents said no to this, so what can I do that they haven't forbidden?* Enter the cell phone.

When Logan was in the sixth grade, those 1-900 teen chat lines were all the rage. Logan and her friends used to call them and "talk" to strangers on the phone. And by *talk*, we mean they described their bodies (i.e., lie about the size of their breasts) and discuss sex. Today, Logan would be horrified if transcripts of those conversations were made public. Thankfully, her preteen verbal-sexual experimentation will never come back to haunt her. But that doesn't mean she didn't do it.

Logan was attempting to express her own sexuality back then, in a presumably "safe" way. The same adolescent rationale applies to sexting. How do you show someone that you like them without doing something that compromises your parents' values? (We know, we know—sexting isn't on a parent's list of appropriate behaviors, but unless you are clear with your kids, they won't instinctively understand that.)

So ask your daughter why she did it. Chances are, she may not be able to express her motivation, but you just got a glimpse of it. Now, on the other hand, if her boyfriend asked her to do it, that's a different story altogether. People who love and respect their boyfriends or girlfriends never ask them to do anything that compromises their safety or their values, no matter what. If your daughter did this to appease a partner, it is time to reevaluate that relationship.

There is yet another issue at play here, and that is whether or not you should notify the boy's parents. In the case of sexting, which has legal implications, the answer is yes. It is better to deal with this early on, before it turns into something bigger.

⑥ Is sexting illegal?

Sexting is legally defined as the act of sending and/or receiving sexually explicit text messages through a phone, computer, or other electronic device. The messages often contain an attachment with an explicit photo or video, sometimes involving the sender, other times featuring friends or acquaintances. It's an act that often involves teenagers, usually high school students, though younger students and adults are also involved in sexting.

Many states have begun criminalizing sexting because of safety and privacy concerns. At least fourteen states, including New York, Pennsylvania, Ohio, Indiana, and Virginia, have passed some type of sexting law, and many more are introducing antisexting statutes into their criminal legislation. By the time you read this, the number of states with criminal laws involving sexting will likely have grown.

If the subject matter of the message involves a person under the age of eighteen, it is possible that the recipient of the message will be charged with possession of child pornography. If the recipient passes along the message, they can be charged with distribution of pornographic materials.

It may seem harmless or even funny to your child to forward these messages, but the penalty of doing so can be pretty severe: fines, criminal records, mandatory counseling, and potential jail time.

We highly recommend discussing these issues with your children before you hand them a phone or electronic device of their own.

The FBI offers this advice to young people:

∵ Think about the consequences of taking, sending, or forwarding a sexual picture of yourself or someone else underage. You could get kicked off sports teams, face humiliation, lose educational opportunities, and even get in trouble with the law.

∵ Never take images of yourself that you wouldn't want everyone—your classmates, your teachers, your family, and your employers—to see.

∵ Before hitting SEND, remember that you cannot control where this image may travel. What you transmit to a boyfriend or girlfriend easily could end up with their friends, and *their* friends, and *their* friends.

:• If you forward a sexual picture of someone underage, you are as responsible for this image as the original sender is. You could face child-pornography charges, go to jail, and have to register as a sex offender.

:• Report any nude pictures you receive on your cell phone to an adult you trust. Do not delete the message. Instead, get your parents or guardians, teachers, and school counselors involved immediately.

7 My daughter's friends are engaging in "beauty contests" on Instagram. I think it's awful. How can I convey that to my daughter?

Confiscate her iPhone, hit it with a hammer, and move to Amish country. Maybe that was over the top, but, in all seriousness, it is that type of online behavior that makes us want to escape our current lives and move to an island in the middle of nowhere with no Wi-Fi.

If you are unfamiliar with Instagram, it is a photo-sharing medium that allows people to post images that others can "follow" and comment on. This user-driven content, like so much else online, affords users a great deal of anonymity and, in some cases, a false sense of security. Instagram at its best is a photo-sharing site; at its worst, it is yet another medium for online bullying. Beauty contests (identified by the hashtag #beautycontest) are created by people posting their pictures on Instagram and waiting for the comments to roll in. If someone (typically a girl) gets too many negative comments, she is eliminated. Elimination is public, indicated by a red X over the girl's face. This does what you would imagine: damages a girl's self-esteem and links her self-worth and value with her face and body.

We would never allow our own children to take part in any way in these beauty contests. How you can monitor this activity on top of everything else you have to do is a fair question, but sometimes it's simply a matter of proactively discussing Instagram and the dreaded #beautycontest with your kids.

Consider posing the following questions to your daughters (and sons):

:• How would you feel if someone said you were unattractive?

:• How would you feel if *many* people said you were unattractive?

:• How would you feel if someone said you were pretty?

:• Why should people care what a stranger online says about them?

However, it's not just Instagram and these beauty contests that you have to worry about—by the time you read this, there will be fifty more types of competitions, eliminations, and apps just waiting to make your child feel judged and insecure. Ask.fm is the latest in a series of other less-than-lovely social-networking sites. As we write this book, there's a story trending in the news about a teenager who took her own life because she was the victim of hateful and cruel comments on this site. While it seems harmless at first glance, Ask.fm is a question-and-answer app that boasted fifty-seven million users in June 2013, is adding two hundred thousand members per day, and is spreading like wildfire through middle schools and high schools, as quickly as Instagram, Snapchat, Kik, and Vine. Not sure what some of these are? You probably will at some point in the near future.

But we digress. Ask.fm's primary users are under the age of eighteen. On the site, they ask their friends or acquaintances anonymous questions, ranging from "What's your favorite subject?" to "Who's your favorite teacher?" to "Who do you have a crush on?" Seems harmless, but, unfortunately, this has become a forum that exposes some kids to malicious postings, racial slurs, sexual taunts or insults, and personal assaults.

Local middle-school administrators in Jena's school district have already warned parents about the inappropriate use of certain social-media apps. This is just another reason why we need to be "plugged in" as parents, so that we can be aware of how to navigate what's new and what's coming down the pike in this never-ending stream of new technology. Even if your child tries to tell you that are apps that make text or photo streams disappear after a few seconds, such as Snapchat, you can tell them that there are always ways to get around those safeguards. Nothing is as safe as it seems, which means we need to be smarter and savvier.

We are not saying no to technology in general—it affords us incredible opportunities to connect to one another in ways we could not possibly have imagined. We rely on it daily, too. However, it is too easy for some of these new sites to do more harm than good in the hands of young people (or adults) who use them in abusive ways.

8 Do you believe in parental controls for the computer?

That depends on which one of us you're asking. (You didn't think we would always agree, did you?) Jena believes in parental controls for the computer. She feels they can offer peace of mind to parents who cannot monitor the amount of inappropriate or violent content their child may be exposed to by simply browsing. Logan, on the other hand, isn't too keen on parental controls. As a sex educator she knows how easy it is for good information about sex and sexuality to disappear simply because a search term contains s-e-x. Her friends don't get half of her emails to them because the word *sexologist* is in her digital signature.

All that aside, parental controls is basically a fancy name for a large selection of software that offers anything from content filtering and blocking options to web-browser monitoring. While it may give you some peace of mind, let us be perfectly clear: If you do decide to turn on your computer's filters or purchase additional software, remember that nothing can ensure total online safety for your child. While parental controls certainly allow parents greater control over their child's Internet activities, there are many stories about tech-savvy children who can bypass the software or partial protection over newly evolved media. And let's face it, if your kids have grown up in the technological age, even the youngest among them is far savvier than any of us.

As with all of the other matters that arise during puberty, communication is key here, too. Parental controls may be a supplement to your family's strategies at home, but you have to lay the groundwork for smart computer skills. We think the best approach to keeping our kids safe online is to work with them to establish a safety policy that they can get on board with. Our experience suggests that the most effective approach to keeping kids safe online is not to make grandiose proclamations and rules, but rather to work side by side with children to create guidelines that they can understand and abide by. Our rules may not align with yours, but you and any parenting partner you have must be on the same page about this subject, so discuss it on your own before you broach it with your child.

9 I saw in my computer's web-browsing history that my son and two of his friends were looking at porn sites last weekend. Should I address this situation?

Part of being a parent means initiating not-so-comfortable conversations; pornography can certainly be one of those if you're not prepared. First thing first: It is not surprising that teens (even young teens) are curious about sex.

If you think back to your own childhood, you can probably remember your first pornography experience. When Logan was in elementary school, her friend found her father's stash of BDSM magazines. By sixth grade, Logan and her friends were trying to watch the Playboy Channel through the static on her friend's cable television. What we're trying to say is that being fascinated by (or even interested in seeing) pornography is very normal. Sure, our children's access to it is greater than ever before, and we should be cognizant of that, but we shouldn't panic if our kids have seen pornography. Instead, we should ask them to think about what they saw and whether they have questions about it, and then we need to teach them to be pornographically literate.

What does it mean to be pornographically literate?

:• Knowing that sex in pornography is not representative of sex in an average relationship

:• Understanding that the majority of pornography does not show any type of safer-sex activity (use of condoms, dental dams, etc.)

:• Being aware that participants do not negotiate their desires and boundaries before engaging in any type of sex—i.e., they do not model the conversations that should take place before engaging in any physically intimate behavior

⑩ My daughter just asked me why Kim Kardashian is so successful even though she has a sex tape. How would you respond?

Before we share our response, our immediate reaction is that the world is a frightening place. And it's not just Kim Kardashian. Farrah Abraham, star (if you can call her that) of MTV's *Teen Mom*, "performed" in her own sex tape with adult-film star James Deen in 2013. The day the films was released, more than twice as many people viewed it in the first twelve hours than they did Kim's taped escapade in the same time frame. Sure, the online distribution system has changed, and more people have access to pornography than they did a few years ago. However, the real issue for us is that the fame and financial success these women have garnered through their sexual activity make our job as parents significantly more difficult.

Please be assured that this is not an indictment of people who work in the adult-entertainment industry; rather, it's a commentary on how women's potential for notoriety seems to be dependent upon their bodies and what they do with them sexually.

We recommend that you turn the question back to your daughter. Ask her versions of the following questions:

:• Why do *you* think Kim Kardashian is so successful?

:• What would you want to become famous for?

:• What effect do you think Kim and Farrah have on young women and men?

Our culture isn't changing anytime soon, but at least this conversation will help you to identify where your teen's values lie.

6

Tobacco, Alcohol, and Other Drugs

Y OUR YOUNGEST SON takes medication for attention deficit hyperactivity disorder (ADHD), and your older son recently asked if he could try a few pills. Apparently, his friends have told him that the medication will make him perform better on tests. Some of his female friends have taken the pills to lose weight. He tells you, "It's a wonder drug. Everyone else is taking it before school. Why can't I? It's legal, after all."

Therein lies the problem. How do you send the right message to your kids about substance abuse, when their siblings are taking prescription medication and their parents come home from work and pour a glass of wine (or two)? (We are by no means suggesting that your cocktails aren't well deserved, but they can send mixed messages.) As your children move from adolescence to young adulthood, they will encounter a variety of these lifestyle choices. Add some peer pressure, and things get even more complicated.

Studies have shown that during developmental transitions such as puberty, children are likely to experiment with tobacco, alcohol, and other substances. The pressure is compounded by the fact that during this period, kids are searching for an increasing sense of independence.

Just being an adolescent may be a key risk factor not only in experimenting with different substances but also in using them without worrying about the consequences. Prescription-drug use is a perfect example. Many kids feel that these substances are less dangerous than other drugs because they are legal. Unfortunately, the use of prescription medications is way up among middle- and high-school students in the United States. Students are using drugs to stay awake to study, to lose weight, and just to get high, without recognizing their real dangers. In this chapter, we will highlight some of the more popular drugs and educate parents about how to spot signs of abuse and get help for their children.

As important as it is to explain the health effects of substance abuse on children, it's even more important for both children and parents to understand the power of peer pressure. If everyone else is taking Ritalin before the PSATs, will your kid do as well on the test if he doesn't? And what about the story Jena heard on her local news in June 2012, about a mother who hosted a party where she served alcohol to high-school students but thought that was acceptable because the kids were under adult supervision? The presence of a few middle school children didn't seem to bother her either, but other parents in her community were outraged.

We've spoken to many people who complain that other parents, rather than kids themselves, pose the biggest problems during the teen years. Some mothers and fathers try to recapture their youth by living vicariously through their kids; some want their children to be "popular" or "cool" at any cost. One woman even told us that she'd rather her daughter be a bully than a "loser." (We know how you feel—it made us sick, too.) Another dad said, "Everyone drinks. What's the big deal?" (His fourteen-year-old daughter got so intoxicated before a school event that she threw up outside.)

Add to that the issue of "absentee parenting," which describes what another father told us: Parents in his community were rarely home to supervise their children's parties. In the case he described, a group of ninth-grade boys had free rein over a basement refrigerator filled with beer. One boy, who had never had an alcoholic beverage, drank with his friends and passed out in the basement, and when his parents called his cell phone to check in, no one picked up. (No one picked up the house phone, either.) Not surprisingly, his parents panicked, drove to the house, and took their son home.

Unfortunately, these stories are not a rarity. Rather, they seem to be part of a disturbing trend that stems from more-permissive parenting and the acceptance that experimentation will always happen. In some ways, this is true: it *is* in our nature to experiment. The key for all of us, then, is to understand how we can manage or minimize the risks that our children take.

1 **My husband offered my thirteen-year-old son a sip of beer to show him that it doesn't taste good. I'm furious. Who is right?**

The short answer is, both of you or neither of you, depending on how you look at it. We subscribe to two different schools of thought on this subject. Many of us have heard the theory that the American obsession with forbidding alcohol consumption until the age of twenty-one is what causes kids in the United States to rebel and abuse alcohol. Europeans, we've been told, aren't as crazy about alcohol, and as a result, their teenagers are much more responsible around alcohol and have fewer abuse issues. That's probably what your husband in this scenario was thinking (at least, we hope it is).

Researchers from Yale University have studied this idea in depth and have disproved the theory that letting underage children sip alcoholic beverages at home somehow leads to more responsible drinking in adulthood. Their research actually associated alcohol use from earlier ages with heavier drinking later on and with more negative consequences.

If you look at the global community as a whole, teen substance abuse is not unique to the United States. Kids from all over the world are consuming large quantities of alcohol. According to a Narconon International endorsed study, young people who start abusing any addictive substance before the age of fifteen are at least six times more likely to wind up with a substance-abuse problem.

That brings us to the second school of thought, which Jena endorses: Banning alcohol in underage drinkers will not turn them into alcoholics later in life. Though it may seem harmless to offer your underage son or daughter a sip of alcohol, Jena sides with the mom on this one.

Logan's philosophy is quite different. She believes that it is important for children to know that alcohol can be part of a larger culinary experience and culture. We frequently see alcohol consumed in mass quantities, and binge drinking seems to show up in the news every fall. Logan thinks that young people should know that (as with everything in life), there are ways to do things smartly.

Now, what if your child asks why they can't have more than a sip? That's fairly easy: Stick with the facts. It is illegal (in the United States) for people to consume alcohol if they are younger than twenty-one. Also, a teen's brain and body cannot process alcohol the way an adult body can. Research studies point to scientists' discovery that the parts of the brain responsible for controlling impulses and planning ahead—features often characterized as "adult behavior"—are among the last to mature in the brains of teens and young adults. Therefore, teenagers may have a harder time understanding the full range of consequences from their choices regarding alcohol. In addition, their tolerance to the effects of alcohol is often much lower than that of an adult. Both of these factors make consuming alcohol riskier for young people.

We all know that our children sometimes make decisions that we are not proud of or that go against everything we have taught

them. If that happens, we need to have contingency plans in place.
For example:

- Ask your child to call home (at any hour) before they get
  into a car with a drunk or drugged driver—no questions
  asked (until the next morning).

- Ask your child to use a buddy system at all times. The
  buddy can call your home at any time, too, for any reason,
  no questions asked. We've spoken to numerous parents
  who serve as an emergency contact for their friend's children; for whatever reason, calling a best friend's mom or
  dad seems more palatable for certain kids.

If you do allow underage drinking, discussing limits is essential. Some kids will drink no matter what, but teaching them to
recognize their own limits, so that they can cut themselves off before they are too intoxicated to make good choices, can save their
life. Although we've already mentioned drunk driving, we think
it's worth bringing up again, as it's one of the most obvious ways
in which impaired function can be fatal. By the same token, encouraging your children to make good decisions about driving or
getting into a car with an intoxicated driver can be lifesaving.

Even though we may disagree about the answer to the original
question, we want to make sure that we are universally clear about
the motivations behind teen drinking. People drink for all kinds of
different reasons: to escape reality, to legitimize feelings (sexual or
otherwise) or to be part of a group. No matter who our children

are, we need them to own their feelings so that they don't rely on alcohol or drugs in order to feel good about themselves.

There is another issue that colors this entire conversation. It is always important to (try to) be on the same page as your parenting partner, if you have one. And if you disagree, you should deal with these issues before they come up, not after you've already made a decision or acted on it. Presenting a united front is incredibly important when it comes to issues like these. Otherwise, your child can become confused and/or dismiss whichever decision they don't agree with—and that's never a good scenario.

❷ My son asked me what will happen to his brain if he drinks. What should I say?

Our philosophy is that you should always be truthful, so give him the facts. We strongly believe that knowledge is power. Remember that 1980s commercial with the egg in the frying pan: "This is your brain on drugs"? It used to scare the crap out of Jena. She wondered if the egg ever bounced back. Which led to many more questions: What if you took only a sip of alcohol or a puff of something? What if, like Bill Clinton, you didn't inhale? Was that egg doomed forever?

The goal is never to scare your children (which tends to backfire), but you don't need to dance around the subject either. Give it to them straight. And if you need a refresher, here it is:

Alcohol definitely affects the brain. Depending on how much and how often a person drinks, it can cause:

:• Nausea and vomiting

:• Difficulty walking

:• Blurred vision

:• Slurred speech

:• Slowed reaction times

:• Impaired memory

:• Poor decision making

:• Inability to consent

Some of these reactions are detectable even after only one or two drinks and quickly disappear when the drinking stops. But studies have shown that people who drink heavily over a long period of time may experience persistent brain impairment. The long-term effects of alcohol on the brain are one of the most heavily researched topics in alcohol studies today. The results of these studies remain to be seen, but the take-home message is the same: Alcohol has both short-term and long-term effects on the brain and on cognitive functioning.

③ My daughter thinks it's okay to "borrow medication" if a family member or friend has a prescription for it, because it's not an illegal drug. Can you help me explain why this is not okay?

We can't tell you how common this scenario is. While we were writing this book, Jena spoke to a woman whose son had just been diagnosed with ADHD. The woman's daughter went to a doctor's appointment with her brother and heard the physician talk about the known side effects of his ADHD medication—including appetite suppression. (You can imagine where this is going.) The woman's daughter asked if she could borrow her brother's medication to lose weight. When this mother said absolutely not, her daughter couldn't understand why: not only was it a legal drug, but several of her friends were already using these types of pills to stay awake to study for exams.

We've all heard the stories on the news (and sometimes in our own communities) about kids raiding their parents' medicine cabinets and trying painkillers, antidepressants, and even heart medication to experiment or just to see what those pills do. The reasoning may be fairly simple: *If it's legal and a doctor prescribed it, it must be okay.* However, not only is this justification faulty, but it can also be dangerous.

Prescription medications for conditions like ADHD, anxiety, depression, or pain management help the people they are prescribed for in very specific ways. They are prescribed, or should be, after a doctor consults the patient's complete medical history and conducts a thorough physical exam. Every medication has pros and cons, side effects, and possible negative interactions with other medications, all of which is taken into consideration when a doctor fills out a prescription. It is a highly regulated process.

Taking prescription medication that *isn't* prescribed for you is not only dangerous but also illegal. We've heard many stories in the news about girls and boys popping three to four Adderall pills (the medication used to treat ADHD) at a time to stay awake or to lose weight. As this is definitely not the recommended dosage, many young people end up in the hospital. If not taken as prescribed, these pills can cause headaches, nausea, vomiting, a racing heart, high blood pressure, tremors, seizures, and even death.

Give your daughter the information and all the details, and impress upon her the seriousness of this issue. If necessary, you can do some research on your own, but keep in mind that information that is completely fear-based can backfire. And remember that when it comes to legality, your daughter is absolutely wrong.

4 **I overheard my daughter's friends talking about how marijuana is not as unhealthy as cigarettes. Is that true?**

Your daughter's friends probably heard this story on the news. And, whether you like it or not, there is some truth behind what they're saying. But it's not that simple, so let's just get the facts out of the way first. A study published in the *Journal of the American*

Medical Association in 2012 analyzed tobacco and marijuana use among more than five thousand people and found that occasional marijuana use does not appear to have long-term adverse effects on lung function, compared with tobacco.

However, marijuana is not without its own risks. Research findings from a 2010 study from the National Institute on Drug Abuse revealed that marijuana users who began in adolescence showed a profound deficit in connections in regions of the brain responsible for learning and memory. Marijuana can cause all sorts of physiological and psychological effects, including rapid heartbeat, increased blood pressure, red eyes, dry mouth, increased appetite, and slow reaction time. It can also cause paranoia, anxiety, memory loss, depression, and a distorted sense of time—not to mention that it's illegal in most states.

Our kids are exposed to media stories from every outlet, every angle, in ways we didn't have access to as children, so it can be challenging for parents to address every story or every study that your child may hear. When the Newtown shooting occurred in December 2012, the news was everywhere. Before Jena had the chance to discuss the tragedy and aftermath with her seven-year-old son, he had learned about the event from an older friend on the bus, who had an iPhone in his backpack. Pictures of assault rifles and the shooter were everywhere. While the nation mourned, many parents across the country grappled with what and how much information to share with their kids—some of whom knew more details than their parents.

When logging on to a computer, your child may be inundated with news headlines, video clips, and sex scandals in a matter of seconds, without giving you the opportunity to catch your breath— let alone figure out how to address any questions or issues that arise. But we recommend keeping the lines of communication open at all times, especially if your child has read or seen something they would like to discuss.

In this example, there's nothing wrong with validating what your daughter's friends have said, but it's also important to emphasize that even though occasional pot smoking may not result in a noticeable decrease in lung function, inhaling anything into the lungs over a long period of time is never healthy. Marijuana use and all of its negative health-related effects should certainly be discussed and discouraged.

But you know what's coming next, right? You child is going to ask you if *you've* ever tried pot. Don't start sweating yet—think about it first. Is your child asking because it will give her "permission" to smoke pot, too? Is it because her friends have been discussing their parents' former lives? You don't have to tell the truth in entirety, but it is crucial to put the answer into context for your daughter. Part of the problem with illegal drugs today is that they are often combined with many other dangerous substances. You may think you're smoking marijuana, but it could contain something you would not be willing to try under any circumstance.

Some parents feel uncomfortable or hypocritical telling their kids not to smoke pot because they've used it themselves. We believe in honesty, so if your child asks you directly whether you've used marijuana, we recommend that you fess up. (Don't just blurt it out, though; first, you need to find out your child's motivation for asking this question. That will help you decide how much to share.) If you do tell them, try not to make your marijuana use seem like part of the "good old glory days." Remember, we had less information back then; now, we know more about the outcomes of drug use. Explain to them how much or how little you knew, why you made the particular decision you did, and what you hope for them. Your values are key to this conversation.

But this isn't always about our past. The increasing availability and legality of medicinal marijuana mean that you, your friends, or your relatives may now use it in some states. There is a chance that your children know this already; in this case, the same rules with respect to honesty apply. According to a 2013 study published in the *New England Journal of Medicine*, more than three in four doctors approve of medicinal marijuana. It has been shown to relieve pain, improve mood, and increase appetite in patients who use it. Research supports honesty as well: A 2009 study from the Hazelden addiction treatment center in Minnesota found that many teenagers believe parental forthrightness about drug and alcohol use had a positive influence on them.

5 **How can we tell my daughter not to smoke cigarettes,
when my husband does?**

First, you can acknowledge the obvious hypocrisy of this discussion. Call it what it is (because if you have savvy children, they'll figure it out anyway), by saying something like, "We know that you're probably confused by this conversation because your dad smokes. It is not something that we are proud of. It is a very bad and obviously unhealthy habit that he cannot quit, as much as he'd like to. Are we being hypocritical? Yes, we are, but that's because you have a choice to be healthy now. Parents don't always make the best decisions, but we can help our children make the right ones."

You can also explain that the real problem with your daughter's trying cigarettes is that the origins of addiction are often unclear, and the progression from social smoking to full-blown nicotine addiction can be insidious. We've seen the same thing happen with bulimia: some girls have told us they thought occasional vomiting after meals was no big deal, until they started purging on a regular basis and then could no longer control it. Addiction is addiction; it's a slippery slope that can be difficult to get off once you've started down it.

6 **My underage son was invited to a party where the parents will be home but will be serving beer. All of his friends are going, so of course he wants to go, too. I'm confused; I don't want him to feel left out.**

None of us hopes for our kids to be friendless, but this is one where you need to trust your gut. We get that your son wants to be one of the gang. Who doesn't? But this isn't even a teen issue; this is definitely a parenting issue, one that you can absolutely address with these parents. In many states, hosting a party with underage drinking is illegal, even if the host parents let everyone know what will be going on in their house. So in some cases, this isn't just a group of teens experimenting with beer; this is parent-sanctioned drinking.

One survey of US teens, published in the *Journal of Adolescent Health* in 2004, found that adults play an important role in teen drinking. Adult-supervised settings for alcohol use resulted in higher levels of harmful alcohol consequences. When parents supply alcohol, the message is clear: Drinking is okay, even though it is illegal. Other studies have shown that adolescents who are allowed to drink at home drink more heavily outside the home. On the other hand, in homes where parents have specific rules against underage drinking and drink responsibly themselves, studies have shown that children are less likely to drink heavily. Our behavior as parents makes a big difference in our child's future drinking behavior and understanding of what we allow inside and outside our homes. So think like a teen for a moment: What would your teen think if you had a drink and then got into the driver's seat of a car? It's not that you couldn't legally do it, but it could certainly send the wrong message to your child. So, sure, have wine with dinner or a cocktail after work, but remember, your kids are always watching.

If you happen to be a parent who is hosting a party where alcohol will be served, there are significant risks involved for you, too. Accidents happen more often when alcohol is a factor, and parents can be held responsible for any accident that happens as a result of underage drinking in their home. Even if they provide only one drink, adults are still liable for all of the drinks that a minor may consume—and it is impossible to pinpoint the one drink that may have pushed a person over their limit and caused an accident. As a result, host parents can be both criminally and civilly liable.

And that's not all. Those parents are also liable for any consequences caused or suffered by any underage drinker, such as sex offenses or assault—even if the person is no longer at their home. (While we don't want to come off as overly dramatic, it is crucial that you understand how severe the consequences may be. The 2012 rape of a girl in Steubenville, Ohio, happened at a party where parent-sanctioned alcohol use occurred.) Any way you look at it, attending this party (or hosting it) is a bad idea.

7 My son is worried that his best friend is taking drugs. He wants to help, but should he get involved? If so, what can he do?

It is admirable that your son wants to help his friend. Sometimes just calling attention to the issue is enough to encourage someone to get help; other times, it's not. Ultimately, the person who is using a substance has to want to get help, and that means he has to accept that there is a problem in the first place. Your son can open the door, but it's his friend who needs to walk through it.

People have many reasons for experimenting with drugs. Some try in hopes of having a good time or because their friends are doing it; some use substances to improve athletic performance or to relieve stress, anxiety, or depression. Some of this may already be predestined. If your son's friend has a family history of addiction, he may be more likely to become addicted to a substance, so helping this boy lies partly in identifying why his behavior has started to begin with.

If your son isn't sure that his friend has a drug problem, he can look for the following signs:

:• Bloodshot eyes or dilated pupils (though some kids use eye drops to try to hide these symptoms)

:• Skipping class

:• Declining grades or school performance

:• Acting differently (isolated, angry, depressed, with-
   drawn, etc.)

:• Dropping an old group of friends for a new one

:• Loss of interest in old activities

:• Stealing money or valuables

Drug experimentation isn't the same thing as a drug problem,
but if your son's friend's drug use is causing issues for him—at
school, at home, or both—it is likely that he already needs some
help. Early use is a risk factor for abuse and addiction, and the risk
of abuse increases if someone using substances is going through
a transitional time, such as a move, a divorce, or a death in the
family.

It is important for your son's friend to know that your son is
concerned about him, but your son also needs to be prepared for
a negative or angry response. This friend may feel as if your son
is betraying him in some way (though your son is definitely doing
the right thing—and we recommend stressing that point when you
advise him). If you need some outside assistance with moving this
process along, you might encourage your son to talk to his school
counselor.

concluding thoughts

S O THERE YOU have it: our parental road map to guide you through adolescence while maintaining your sanity and sense of humor. Sure, we may be doctors, but we are mothers first. While this time can be exciting, and simultaneously exhausting, hopefully you can embrace it with an open mind and an open heart. Trust your instincts and know that we will be nearby, cheering from the sidelines.

sources

CHAPTER 1

Biro, F. M., et al. "Pubertal Assessment Method and Baseline
Characteristics in a Mixed Longitudinal Study of Girls."
Pediatrics 126, no. 3 (2010): 583–90.

CHAPTER 2

Abma, J. C., et al. "Teenagers in the United States: Sexual
Activity, Contraceptive Use, and Childbearing: National Survey
of Family Growth 2006–2008." *Vital and Health Statistics* 23,
no. 30 (2010).

Alan Guttmacher Institute. "U.S. Teenage Pregnancy Statistics:
Overall Trends, Trends by Race and Ethnicity, and State-by-State
Information," January 2010.

Applied Research and Consulting LLC. Liz Claiborne Inc. study
of teens 13–17, spring 2000.

Elfenbein, D. S., and M. E. Felice. "Adolescent Pregnancy." In *Nelson Textbook of Pediatrics*, 19th ed. Edited by R. M. Kliegman, et al. Philadelphia: Saunders Elsevier, 2011.

Herbenick, D., Schick, V., Reece, M., Sanders, S. A., Smith, N., Dodge, B. and Fortenberry, J. D. (2013), "Characteristics of Condom and Lubricant Use Among a Nationally Representative Probability Sample of Adults Ages 18–59 in the United States." *Journal of Sexual Medicine*, 10: 474–483. doi: 10.1111/jsm.12021.

Jones, R. K. *Beyond Birth Control: The Overlooked Benefits of Oral Contraceptive Pills*. New York: Guttmacher Institute, 2011.

Kohler, P. K., L. E. Manhart, and W. E. Lafferty. "Abstinence-Only and Comprehensive Sex Education and the Initiation of Sexual Activity and Teen Pregnancy." *Journal of Adolescent Health* 42 (2008), 344–51.

Martinez, G., et al. "Teenagers in the United States: Sexual Activity, Contraceptive Use, and Childbearing, 2006–2010," *Vital and Health Statistics* 23, no. 31 (2011).

National Health Statistics Reports. "Prevalence and Timing of Oral Sex with Opposite-Sex Partners Among Females and Males Aged 15–24 Years: United States, 2007–2010," no. 56, August 16, 2012.

National Teen Dating Abuse Healthline, in coordination with Liz Claiborne Inc. "Tween and Teen Dating Violence and Abuse Study," February 2008.

Pew Research Center. Internet & American Life Project, 2011.

Richtel, Matt. "Young, in Love and Sharing Everything, Including a Password." *New York Times*, January 17, 2012.

University of Texas Health Science Center at Houston. "Middle School Youth as Young as 12 Engaging in Risky Sexual Activity." *Science Daily*, April 10, 2009.

CHAPTER 3

Bateman, Helen Vrailas. "Sense of Community in the School: Listening to Students' Voices." In *Psychological Sense of Community: Research, Applications, and Implications*. Edited by Adrian T. Fisher, Chris C. Sonn, and Bryant J. Bishop. New York: Kluwer Academic/Plenum Publishers, 2002.

Brown, B. Bradford. "Peer Groups and Peer Cultures." In *At the Threshold: The Developing Adolescent*. Edited by Shirley S. Feldman and Glen R. Elliott. Cambridge, MA: Harvard University Press, 1990.

Brown, G. K., et al. "Cognitive therapy for the prevention of suicide attempts: a randomized controlled trial." *Journal of the American Medical Association* 294, no. 5 (2005): 563–70.

Gould, M. S., et al. "Youth Suicide Risk and Preventive Interventions: A Review of the Past 10 Years." *Journal of the American Academy of Child and Adolescent Psychiatry* 24, no. 4 (2003): 386–405.

Greydanus, D. *The Complete and Authoritative Guide: Caring For Your Teenager*. Washington, DC: The American Academy of Pediatrics, 2003.

Perkins, H. W., et al. "Using Social Norms to Reduce Bullying: A Research Intervention Among Adolescents in Five Middle Schools." *Group Processes & Intergroup Relations*, 14, no. 5 (2011): 703–22.

U.S. Public Health Service. "National Strategy for Suicide Prevention: Goals and Objectives for Action." Rockville, MD: USDHHS, 2001.

CHAPTER 4

Camargo Carlat, D. J. "Review of Bulimia in Males." *American Journal of Psychiatry* 154, no. 8 (1997): 1127–32.

Gurian, A. "How to Raise Girls with Healthy Self-Esteem." NYU Child Study Center, June 2012.

Hudson, J. I., et al. "The Prevalence and Correlates of Eating Disorders in the National Comorbidity Survey Replication." *Biological Psychiatry* 61, no. 3 (2007): 348–58.

Michael, S. L., et al. "Parental and Peer Factors Associated with Body Image Discrepancy Among Fifth-Grade Boys and Girls." *Journal of Youth and Adolescence*, January 19, 2013.

National Eating Disorders Association. Fact sheet, 1991.

Sutin, A. R., and A. Terracciano. "Perceived Weight Discrimination and Obesity." *PLoS One* 8, no. 7 (2013): e70048. doi:10.1371/journal.pone.007048.

University of Bristol. The Avon Longitudinal Study of Parents and Children (ALSPAC), (also known as "Children of the 90s"), 1991–present.

CHAPTER 6

Foley, K. L., et al. "Adults' Approval and Adolescents' Alcohol Use." *Journal of Adolescent Health* 35, no. 4 (2004): 7–26.

Morean, M. "Both early alcohol use and early intoxication can herald trouble for college students." *Alcoholism: Clinical and Experimental Research*, November 2012.

Morean, M. E., and W. R. Corbin. "Subjective response to alcohol: a critical review of the literature." *Alcoholism: Clinical and Experimental Research* 24, no. 3 (2010): 385–95.

National Institute on Alcohol Abuse and Alcoholism. "Understanding the Impact of Alcohol on Human Health and Well-Being." Fact sheets, September 2012.

Pletcher, M. J., et al. "Association Between Marijuana Exposure and Pulmonary Function Over 20 Years." *Journal of the American Medical Association* 307, no. 2 (2012): 173–81.

Van der Vorst, H., et al. "The Impact of Alcohol-Specific Rules, Parental Norms About Early Drinking and Parental Alcohol Use on Adolescents' Drinking Behavior." *Journal of Child Psychology and Psychiatry* 47, no. 12 (2006): 1299–1306.

Van der Vorst, H., R. C. M. E. Engels, and W. J. Burk. "Do Parents and Best Friends Influence the Normative Increase in Adolescents' Alcohol Use at Home and Outside the Home?" *Journal of Studies on Alcohol and Drugs* 71, no. 1 (2010): 105–14.

index

acknowledgments

THANKS FROM BOTH OF US

There is nothing better than knowing that people believe in a project you're passionate about. This book could not have been published without the support of Krista Lyons, Laura Mazer, Donna Galassi, Natalie Nicolson, Eva Zimmerman, and the entire team at Seal Press. That being said, this book could not have been written without our editor, Annie Tucker. Thank you for taking our two chatty and sometimes wordy personalities and weaving them into something melodic and unified.

And, of course, none of this could have been achieved without our agent, Kathryn Beaumont. You believed in us from the very beginning; we are so very grateful.

THANKS FROM LOGAN

Writing a book can be an arduous task. Having a coauthor can either greatly complicate an already challenging job or make the process blissfully easy. I feel so lucky to have had Jena Wider as my writing partner. You made this experience such a positive one. I could not have asked for a better coauthor, colleague, and friend.

As with most things in my life, I could not (and, quite frankly, would not) have written another book without the unconditional support of my family: my partner in life and love, Lou Cortes; my children, Maverick and Memphis; my parents, Susan and Steven Levkoff; and my sister, Cameron. I fight so strongly to make this world a healthier and happier place because you are all in it.

Of course, a parenting book isn't just about what you put on a page. It comes from hours of talking to your friends, laughing and crying over what life throws at you. To my girls (you know who you are), thank you for providing me with laughter, drinks, and plenty of material to work with.

THANKS FROM JENA

First and foremost, I'd like to thank my coauthor, Logan Levkoff, who is gifted at creating an environment where parents and children feel safe asking any question. I've learned so much from her during this process and can think of no better person to have partnered with to create an invaluable resource for fellow parents.

I'd like to thank my husband, Erez, for his tireless encouragement, his help, and his quiet strength. I'd also like to thank my family—my parents, Barbara and Jerry; my brothers, Todd and Jedd; and my sister-in-law, Danielle—for their constant and unconditional love and support.

To Orly, Ryan, and Piper: wishing you love and peace through your adolescence and beyond—may you always recognize your self-worth and the beauty within, and may you have the confidence to forever be true to yourselves.

about the authors

LOGAN LEVKOFF

Dr. Logan Levkoff is a nationally recognized sexologist, sexuality educator, and author. She is a thought leader in the world of human sexuality, frequently appearing on television shows including *Good Morning America, The Today Show, The Rachael Ray Show, CBS This Morning*, and *Oprah*, and on the Fox News Channel and CNN. Dr. Levkoff is also the host of CafeMom's show *Mom Ed: In the Bedroom*. She is a trusted source for many publications, blogs for *The Huffington Post*, and SheKnows, and is the author of the books *Third Base Ain't What It Used to Be: What Your Kids Are Learning About Sex Today—and How to Teach Them to Become Sexually Healthy Adults* and *How to Get Your Wife to Have Sex with You*.

Dr. Levkoff is dedicated to perpetuating healthy and positive messages about sexuality. She lectures across the country on a wide range of issues. For over a decade, she has been teaching groups of all ages and from a variety of backgrounds. She has designed and implemented sexuality education programs, faculty development, and parent education in many secular and religious independent schools, universities, medical schools, and community organizations. Dr. Levkoff's work with teens and parents has been profiled in numerous publications, including *The New York Times*.

Dr. Levkoff is an AASECT-certified sex educator and serves on AASECT's board of directors. She received her PhD in human sexuality, marriage, and family life education from New York University, and a BA in English and an MS in human sexuality education from the University of Pennsylvania. She has also received certification from the New York Department of Health AIDS Institute. She lives in New York City with her husband, son, and daughter.

JENNIFER WIDER

Jennifer Wider, MD, is a nationally renowned women's health expert, author, and radio host. She has appeared on *The Today Show*, CBS News, *Good Day New York*, Fox News, and news channels 8 and 12 in Connecticut. Dr. Wider is a medical adviser to *Cosmopolitan* magazine and hosts a weekly segment called *Am I Normal?* for Cosmo Radio on SiriusXM. She has also been heard on Bloomberg Radio, Oprah Radio, and WABC-AM talk radio, among many other stations across the country.

Dr. Wider is the author of three other books: *The Savvy Woman Patient*, *The Doctor's Complete College Girls' Health Guide*, and *The New Mom's Survival Guide*. She is a spokesperson and writes a twice-monthly syndicated column for the Society for Women's

Health Research (SWHR), the nation's only nonprofit organization whose mission is to improve the health of all women through
research, education, and advocacy. Her writing has also appeared
in publications including *The New York Times*, *The Wall Street
Journal*, and *Cosmopolitan*, *Glamour*, *SELF*, *Shape*, *Real Simple*,
Weight Watchers, *Prevention*, and *Woman's Day* magazines.

Dr. Wider has been an invited guest lecturer and workshop
presenter at a variety of hospitals, women's centers, high schools,
and colleges across the country. She serves and has served on the
health and medical advisory boards of *Cosmopolitan* magazine,
SWHR, Girls Inc., and SingleEdition.com.

Dr. Wider is a graduate of Princeton University and received
her medical degree from the Mount Sinai School of Medicine in
New York City. She lives in Connecticut with her husband and
three children.

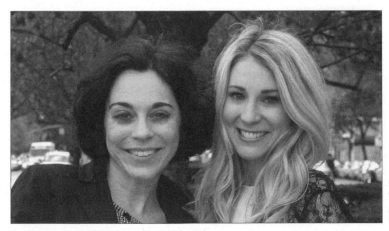

Jennifer Wider (left) and Logan Levkoff (right)

© Erez Salik

selected titles from seal press

The Goodbye Year: Surviving Your Child's Senior Year in High School, by Toni Piccinini. $16.00, 978-1-58005-486-7. Part self-help, part therapy, and completely honest, this sensitive companion is for mothers facing the life-changing transition that occurs when children graduate from high school.

Beautiful You: A Daily Guide to Radical Self-Acceptance, by Rosie Molinary. 16.95, 978-1-58005-331-0. Encourages women, whatever their size, shape, and color, to work toward feeling wonderful about themselves despite today's media-saturated culture.

Gawky: Tales of an Extra Long Awkward Phase, by Margot Leitman. $16.00, 978-1-58005-478-2. Tall girl Margot Leitman's memoir is a hilarious celebration of growing up gangly, a cathartic release of everything awkward girls are forced to endure, and a tribute to a youth that was larger than life.

Reclaiming Our Daughters: What Parenting a Pre-Teen Taught Me About Real Girls, by Karen Stabiner. $14.95, 978-1-58005-213-9. Offers a message of hope and optimism to the parents of adolescent and preadolescent girls.

Girldrive: Criss-Crossing America, Redefining Feminism, by Nona Willis Aronowitz and Emma Bee Bernstein. $19.95, 978-1-58005-273-3. Two young women set out on the open road to explore the current state of feminism in the U.S.

Book by Book: The Complete Guide to Creating Mother-Daughter Book Clubs, by Cindy Hudson. $16.95, 978-1-58005-299-3. Everything moms need to know to start a tradition that builds strong bonds and opens new avenues of conversation with their daughters.

Find Seal Press Online
www.SealPress.com
www.Facebook.com/SealPress
Twitter: @SealPress